ADOLESCENT PATIENTS
IN TRANSITION

Volume I of the McLean Hospital Monograph Series

ADOLESCENT PATIENTS IN TRANSITION

Impact and Outcome of Psychiatric Hospitalization

Mollie C. Grob, S.M.

Judith E. Singer, Ph.D.

With the collaboration of
Golda Edinburg, M.S.S.S.
Richard Longabaugh, Ed.D.
Norbett Mintz, Ph.D.

Including an Introduction by
Francis deMarneffe, M.D.

Behavioral Publications, Inc.
New York

Library of Congress Catalog Number 73-22379
ISBN: 0-87705-137-2
Copyright © 1974 by Behavioral Publications

BEHAVIORAL PUBLICATIONS
72 Fifth Avenue
New York, New York 10011

Printed in the United States of America
456789 987654321

LIBRARY OF CONGRESS CATALOGING
IN PUBLICATION DATA

Grob, Mollie C
    Adolescent patients in transition.

    Bibliography: p. 197
    1. Adolescent psychiatry. 2. Psychiatric hospital care. I.
Singer, Judith E., joint author. II. Title. [DNLM: 1. Adolescent
psychiatry. 2. Hospitalization. 3. Hospitals, Psychiatric—U.S.
WS462 G873a 1974]
RJ503.G76   362.7'8'21

"—the desire signified the victory of his adolescent vigor and sensuality and the first intimation of the mighty forces of life, and the pain signified that the morning peace had been broken, that his soul had left that childhood land which can never be found again. His small ship had barely escaped a near disaster; now it entered a region of new storms and uncharted depths—"

Herman Hesse*

*from *Beneath the Wheel*, published in the United States by Farrar, Straus, and Giroux, 1969.

CONTENTS

LIST OF TABLES

ACKNOWLEDGEMENTS

This study was made possible through the generous funding of an anonymous private donor and, in part, by a General Research Support Grant number 5-501-RR05484-05 from the National Institute of Mental Health

The authors have been particularly fortunate to have had the opportunity to work with several able collaborators: Golda Edinburg, M.S.S.S., Director, Social Work Department, McLean Hospital, functioned as a social work consultant throughout the project; the collaboration of Norbett Mintz, Ph.D., during the early phase of the investigation, was made possible by a Career Development Award from the NIMH, award #Kl-MH-31,212; the collaboration of Richard Longabaugh, Ed.D., currently at Butler Hospital and Brown University, continued to be valuable after he left his position as Director of the Social Science Department at McLean Hospital. We wish to give special acknowledgement to Alfred M. Stanton, M.D. for the interest and consultation he provided during all phases of the study.

We are also indebted to Helen Reinherz, ScD., Director of Research, Simmons College School of Social Work, for her warm support and to the eleven enthusi-

astic second-year graduate students there
who participated in the data collection
and analyses for the second phase of the
study: Shirin H. Bird, Susan W. Brooks,
Louise Enoch, Katharine C. Esty, Bettye
Freeman, Elaine B. Jost, Stacey Lee,
Linda A. Onuska, Lissa Robins, Myra
Schectman, and Paula Berman Sneddon.
    Norma Konstadt assumed major re-
sponsibility for developing the code, and
the long process of coding was made possible with the help of Myrna Chandler
Goldstein, Carole Goldstein, and Sylvia
Hoffman.   The research assistance of Jane
Millikan was invaluable; we are grateful
for her contribution.   Secretaries Barbara
Kavanagh Mallen and Donna Hopwood spent
many long hours patiently typing and re-
typing the manuscripts.
    Without the interest and involvement
of the families who participated, this
project would not have become a reality.
To our own families, special gratitude for
their constant encouragement.

INTRODUCTION

In the early 1960's, psychiatric hospitals were challenged by the special needs of a growing population of new patients - adolescents. Before then, most psychiatric institutions had traditionally treated adults; hospitalization of adolescents was a relatively limited phenomenon.

This was equally true of McLean Hospital. During the 1950's, the hospital gradually began to lower its minimum age requirement for admission. In 1955, six percent of the patients admitted to McLean Hospital were under 21; by 1960-61, the adolescent population had tripled to 18 percent of admissions. This trend of sharply increased percentages of adolescent admissions continued over the decade. In 1970, adolescents comprised more than one-third of the inpatient population.

This phenomenon was not unique to McLean. Other psychiatric hospitals in different parts of the country reported that they also were being flooded by requests to admit adolescents. The 1960's were troubled times for young people, and many sought psychiatric help.

Many hospitals were reluctant to admit adolescents because of uncertainties about the most effective way of handling such patients. The number of adolescent psychiatrists experienced in inpatient treatment of adolescents was extremely limited. There was growing recognition that, as a group, these patients were often very difficult to treat. At McLean, it was decided not to turn away from the difficulties involved but rather to attempt to develop a comprehensive treatment program specifically designed for the adolescent's needs.

The influx of young patients and the commitment to establish such a program raised all kinds of questions and issues. An immediate issue related to the training of psychiatrists who would be responsible for developing adolescent patient units; for example, should the psychiatrist be trained primarily in child psychiatry, or should he be trained primarily in hospital psychiatry, gathering adolescent experience as he worked in the hospital? Because the number of adolescent psychiatrists with inpatient adolescent treatment experience was extremely limited, we had to develop our own training programs. Eventually, this led to the establishment of a residency in adolescent psychiatry at McLean supported by the National Institute of Mental Health.

Another lively issue was that of structuring the best living arrangements for adolescents. Should adolescents be housed in special units, or should they be mixed with older patients? Should the units be sexually integrated or segre-

gated? Decisions about a treatment milieu
best suited to adolescents continued to be
discussed over a period of years. We ex-
perimented with all kinds of arrangements.

The development of our adolescent program coincided with tremendous changes in
society with respect to the young. Even
in more normal times, the period of adolescence has its own particular difficulties.
Adolescence is, by definition, a period of
transition between childhood and adult
life with many psychological and physio-
logical changes taking place. In the early
1960's, not only were adolescents going
through this normal transition, but society
itself was going through a period of transition, a kind of social revolution, if you
will. All mores and values were being
questioned by the young - from politics,
civil rights and the Puritan work ethic to
sexual mores and dress standards. Changing attitudes toward these issues only
served to heighten the normal difficulties
obtaining between generations. These complexities made it very difficult for the
clinical staff to determine what would
constitute a proper setting for treating
adolescents.

There was a major issue, however,
about which we had fairly strong feelings.
The main business of adolescent life, we
reasoned, was education. To deny our
young patients the opportunity to continue
their schooling while hospitalized, would
deprive them of normal adolescent experience. We believed that an educational
hiatus during hospitalization could have
serious repercussions - intellectual, educational, social and economic - later in

the patient's life, perhaps even for the
rest of his life.

Therefore, from the outset, we decided to develop an educational program.
Initially, this took the form of trying to
place a number of adolescent patients in
nearby high schools. For a variety of
reasons, we found this was not very satis-
factory. By the fall of 1961, we had established our own high school on hospital
grounds, in a then unused hospital building; taking the name of that building, it
was called the Arlington School.

We were determined to clearly dis-
tinguish between treatment and education.
The school would be a bona fide educational institution and not simply an extension
of the hospital's clinical program. From
this basic policy decision, flowed certain
other decisions. If we were to establish
a bona fide educational institution, the
faculty should be recruited on the grounds
of their educational experience. We
wanted good teachers. We were not looking
for therapists, counselors, and the like
who would serve as mere adjuncts to the
clinical therapists.

Also, if the school was to provide an
educational experience independent of
therapeutic programs, decisions regarding
courses, educational progress, techniques,
etc. were to be made by the school faculty
independent of the clinical staff. Certainly, there needed to be continuous consultation back and forth between educators
and clinicians, but the clinician would
not recommend courses to provide therapeutic experiences. The school would

function not as a treatment area of Mc-
Lean Hospital, but rather as a "normal-
izing facility" which would try to repli-
cate the function of a school system in
the community as much as possible. Thus,
it could bring a normally expected part
of the larger culture into the mental
hospital which we felt to be particularly
important for younger patients.

These decisions in turn created some
internal problems. The establishment of
Arlington School meant that adolescent
patients would be spending a considerable
portion of their day in school, causing
unavailability during those hours for
clinical services, such as psychotherapy.
Some feeling developed among the clinical
staff that the school, in a sense, was
encroaching on their time for scheduling
clinical activities. There were many
discussions on these and other points, as
clinicians and educators sought that flex-
ibility which would enable them to satisfy
their different needs and roles in a way
that would best help the patient.

The feelings of families of patients
caused other adjustments to be made. They
tended to accept the medical model and the
responsibility of the physician and the
clinical staff in treatment matters. However, the family was more reluctant to
surrender its traditional role of collaboration and participation in the educational process of their children. For many
years, communication about adolescents at
the Arlington School went from the family
to the clinicians to the educators; and
then back from the educators through the
clinical staff to the family. In more

recent years, we have evolved more satis-
factory direct contact between the families and the school, particularly in such
matters as where the student would go
when he graduated from the school.

As we developed our adolescent program, we became more aware of the con-
flicts that are inherent to some degree
in all family-hospital relationships.
Somehow, with the families of adolescent
patients, these problems were brought to
light more clearly. Many patients of
adolescent years are admitted to hospitals
finally as a result of what has come to be
an intolerable conflict between the family
and the child. Many families have reached
their limit of endurance and are often relieved to be able to refer the troubled
child to the care of a hospital.

Initially, the family appears only
too willing to accept the suggestions and
advice of the staff, seeing the hospital
as its ally in dealing with the patient.
However, we began to see that as the patient's treatment began, family feelings
changed. The hospital, for clinical reasons, had to begin taking certain steps
to foster the independence of the adolescent vis-a-vis the family since that, in a
sense, is what the work of treatment and
adolescence is all about. We noticed
quite frequently that, at this stage, the
conflict originally encountered between
patient and family somehow was extended
onto the hospital through the family.
Finding the increased independence of
their adolescent children at times difficult to accept, and resenting the hospital's part in creating that situation,

families often diverted their frustration
from the patient toward the hospital.

   Many disagreements arose between the
family and the hospital as a result of
these underlying feelings and issues, with
repeated complaints of difficulties in
communication. We are still not free of
some of these family-hospital communication
difficulties - nor do we really expect
ever to be fully free of them. But our
experience with families of adolescent
patients over the years has certainly
sensitized us to this problem and helped
us to manage it better.

   The intention of this introduction
has not been to provide a primer on all
the complexities of adolescent treatment,
but rather to present a background perspective against which the purpose and
value of the investigation undertaken
here may be best viewed. I have tried to
show how the development of a comprehensive treatment program for adolescents
produced many stresses and strains upon
the hospital organization as its clinical
staff began moving in an area where relatively little definitive data existed.
While this made us quite open-minded
about taking those actions which would
seem to move us in the direction we wished
to go, we were less certain about our
successes than we had been in treating
many other patient groups. In this spirit,
the decision was made that on-going research and evaluation of the treatment of
the adolescent population be initiated.
We were not only interested in the ulti-
mate results of treatment but wished also
to examine other problems which might lead

to the improvement of our treatment programs, such as family satisfaction and
difficulties in communication.

This work presents the results to
date of a research commitment to hospitalized adolescents; it is illustrative of
continuing efforts at McLean Hospital and
other treatment settings to evaluate their
programs and to adapt them as needed to
new demands imposed by a changing culture
and new developments in the field of
psychiatry.

Francis deMarneffe, M.D.
Director, McLean Hospital
Lecturer in Psychiatry,
  Harvard University

CHAPTER 1

THE STUDY

KAREN, age 16, was admitted to McLean Hospital in May, 1962, having been found in Greenwich Village the previous week. She had called home from there and regaled her parents with the details of her brief stay, including her having been beaten and having been sexually promiscuous. She readily admitted she had "asked for all her trouble". When her parents consulted the psychiatrist to whom she was known (since age 15 for serious school difficulties and unmanagable behavior at home), he recommended an evaluation at McLean. Initially, Karen was resentful of the plan, but finally agreed.

At age 17 1/2, JERRY was admitted to McLean in the late fall of 1961 from a Midwestern university, where he had started his freshman year several weeks earlier. Shortly after arriving at the college, he and his roommate had become involved with two girls, culminating in his becoming quite paranoid about the girl he had dated. He vacillated in his thinking, claiming that he was "a very bad, hopeless person" and then shifting to telling everyone that he was "going to save the world". The family had been called to the college. They returned with Jerry to Boston, consulting a psychiatrist whom the father had known over the years. The psychiatrist recommended hospitalization, and this was easily arranged with Jerry signing in voluntarily. Jerry had had no previous history of psychiatric difficulties.

JOAN was transferred to McLean early in 1963 from another private setting where she had been hospitalized over the previous year. Because of frequent episodes of running back to her mother, and her inability to form a therapeutic alliance, a transfer to an out-of-state hospital had been recommended. At the time of the McLean admission, Joan was 16 1/2 years of age. She had originally been hospitalized because of frequent episodes of running away from home and promiscuous behavior. On at least two occasions she worried that she was pregnant; on another occasion she had contracted venereal disease. Her parents, in desperation, had finally agreed to hospitalize her when all other plans had failed, including boarding school and living with friends of the family.

The advent of an era of increasing numbers of adolescents seeking admission to psychiatric hospitals presented a challenge not only to the skills and resources of the mental health professional, but to his understanding of the nature of the problem itself. Cumulative experience with the young population began to provide an empirical base from which studies could be launched to answer the many persistent questions emerging, such as (1) what were the characteristics of the hospitalized adolescent and his family (2) what factors had led to hospitalization, so unprecedented (3) what was the nature and the effect of the hospitalization (4) how did the adolescent and his family view the experience (5) and, finally, what preadmission, hospital, and post-hospital variables were related to the level of functioning at follow-up? We undertook this investigation in an effort to provide some answers to these questions.

Relatively few published follow-up studies on inpatient adolescent care were available when this study was initiated;[1] several appeared subsequently.[2] Early studies are not strictly comparable because of differences in demographic characteristics, diagnoses of patient populations, and treatment settings; also, criteria for evaluating outcome vary from study to study. Recent studies have had some significant similarities, however, including an increasing methodological sophistication, as well as attempts to correlate pre-hospital, hospital and post-hospital variables. We will not pursue a review of the literature here because it has been so carefully documented in the Hartman et al, Garber, and Gossett et al[3] studies. Some comparison of our results with those appearing in the more recent literature will be made in the final chapters.

Sample

The subjects were all patients between the ages of 13 and 19 who were in residence at McLean Hospital a minimum of three months between 1961 and 1963. There were 36 males and 31 females.

Setting

McLean Hospital is a small, private psycho-analytically oriented psychiatric hospital in Belmont, Massachusetts, a suburb of Boston. Prior to 1960, its patients were almost all adults who tended to come to McLean for traditionally long-term treatment. The atmosphere of the hospital was fairly "upperclass" - patients had private or semi-private rooms in one of 6 buildings, each of which reflected past grandeur. There was a high staff to patient ratio, as well as numerous activities, and essentially a feeling that the patient was given specialized attention.

When adolescents began to arrive, they were mixed with adults in units of 20-25 beds each. Each unit was run by a psychiatrist-administrator; in addition, for the most part, each patient had a psychotherapist.

Procedure

The method of study involved several varied procedures:

1. The Follow-up Interviews. Under the signature of the hospital director, letters were sent to the parents describing the purpose of the study and eliciting their participation. This was followed by a telephone call from the research social worker requesting a personal interview at the hospital, other designated office, the informant's home or place of business. Where possible, former patients were also included as informants. The research social worker offered to visit all families in the northeastern states, using New York City or Boston as a base for families passing through from other outlying areas. Telephone interviews were utilized only in those instances where the respondents were geographically inaccessible. The interview schedules used were comprehensive and had

been coded for later processing. Assess-
ments of the ex-patient's functioning
were made by the respondents and recorded
during the interview. One research social
worker conducted the interviews which were
carried out in a semi-formal manner to
allow for spontaneity.

Interviewing was initiated in 1967 and
continued through 1968, four to ten years
after patient's admission to the hospital.
Of the 62 families interviewd, 15 were
very difficult to locate because of mobility but were all reached through relatives
or friends. Telephone interviews were
necessitated in 20 instances. It was the
interviewer's impression that on the whole,
the telephone interviews were as product-
ive as the personal contacts in providing
the information required, although the
latter seemed to be more rewarding for the
informants. The average interview lasted
approximately two hours.

Follow-up data were obtained for 64 of
the 67 adolescents studied (96 percent)
with 62 families interviewed, and two professional persons for families not available. There were three outright refusals
to participate, two being from families
of deceased adolescents. The largest
single group of respondents seen were
mothers (47 in all); then fathers (37);
and former patients, (24). Two or more
respondents per family were interviewed
for about one half of the sample. There
were 13 refusals on the part of parents to
have the former patient contacted, and two
on the part of their spouses. Reasons
given were usually that the former patient
was better and would not profit from any

discussion of previous hospitalization.
At these times, quite often it turned out
that improvement was relatively recent,
or adjustment was marginal, and parents
were anxious to have the condition better
stabilized. Another group of former patients not interviewed included those with
such disposition as death; jail; out of
town psychiatric hospitalization or residential center; whereabouts unknown; and
geographic inaccessibility.

The level of participation on the part
of families was very high and quite unexpected. At the start of the investigation there was little assurance that the
population to be approached would be responsive to the idea of participating in
"research". Almost all respondents seemed
to appreciate the opportunity to review
the hospital experience and bring the hospital up to date with current information.
They described themselves as highly motivated to cooperate either out of appreci-
ation toward the hospital or as a way of
expressing dissatisfaction with it. Initial resistance on the part of hostile
family members was resolved when the respondent was assured that a candid appraisal of the hospital experience was important to the study. Other frequently expressed reactions to the research included enthusiasm about McLean's concern
in learning about what happened to former
patients and an altruistic interest in the
opportunity to contribute in some way to
future treatment plans. There was evidence to suggest that interviews were
approached by respondents with much thought
beforehand, some going so far as to com-
pile notes. Quite often the first re-

spondent offered to help with making
arrangements for other members of the
family to be seen.

    2.   Preadmission and Hospital Data.
An elaborate code, outlined in Appendix A,
was devised to allow description, in code
form, of the data obtained from the
follow-up interview plus any possibly rel-
avent data on the patients' background and
hospitalization as described in the hospital record. Over 1000 variables were
used to describe each patient from his
parents' background through his birth,
early childhood, school years, adolescence, hospitalization, and life in the
five years after discharge. Some variables were very objective (e.g. sex, religion, education) while some were very
subjective (e.g. school adjustment, parents' attitudes); but, however complex
the variable, each patient was described
quantitatively so as to permit computer
analysis. Because of the difficulty in
expressing qualitative data in such a
form, the code was reworked extensively
with repeated checks for reliability between coders until the coding system
"worked" satisfactorily. One somewhat
unsatisfactory result of the importance
of reliability was the necessity of
allowing the coders to give a rating of
"no data" whenever the data was too am-
biguous to permit reliable codification,
which meant that many variables did not
include data on all patients. On the
other hand, it was fortunate that a
majority of the patients could be described on almost all variables. The
variables on which data sufficient to
permit meaningful analysis were not

obtained are listed in Appendix B.

3. Ratings of Adjustment. Each patient was rated for adjustment at the time
of admission, discharge, and the follow-
up interview. Ratings of GOOD, FAIR, or
POOR were made on the basis of predefined
criteria for adjustment as described in
Appendix C. The coders rated adjustment
with respect to *mental status, adjustment to
mother, adjustment to father, adjustment to peers,*
and *adjustment to work and/or school.* Numerous
reliability checks, followed by extensive
discussion of the criteria for the ratings,
insured that these ratings were reliable
and meaningful. The three raters independently rated each patient on each di-
mension. Whenever a discrepant rating
was obtained, the three discussed the
rating until they reached a unanimous
decision. The data permitted reliable
ratings for most patients on all scales
for the time at admission and follow-up;
however, the data on the patient's adjustment at discharge, as defined by these
criteria, were not clear or available for
most patients on all scales except *mental
status.* Finally, the interviewer made an
additional rating of the ex-patient's
overall adjustment at follow-up.

4. Methods of Analysis. The IBM-370
computer, using Data-text language, was
employed for the data analysis. The first
set of analyses involved frequency distributions of each of the 1072 variables.
The frequency distributions were cross
tabulated by *mental status* ratings: preadmission variables were cross tabulated
by *mental status* at admission, hospitalization variables were cross tabulated by

mental status at discharge, and follow-up
variables were cross tabulated by *mental
status* at follow-up. Follow-up data was
taken from the interviews of the primary
respondents.* Thus, the first round of
analyses permitted an assessment of how
the patients were characterized on each
variable, and how the characterization
was related to whether the patients had
GOOD, FAIR or POOR *mental status*.

These preliminary analyses allowed a
weeding out of irrelevant variables, and
a selection of approximately 250 variables for which data had been obtained on
most patients and on which patients were
distributed in some meaningful way. Variables eliminated included those variables
for which data could not be found for
enough patients (listed in Appendix B) as
well as a host of variables which did not
apply to most patients (e.g. 115 variables
related to "surrogate family", some unus-
ual symptoms, marriages, etc.). The selected variables were next cross-tabulated**

---

*For purposes of data analysis, the
mother was defined as the primary respondent except in instances of some kind
of family disorganization (e.g. loss or
unavailability of mother), in which case
the father was defined as the primary respondent. No important differences were
found between mothers and fathers in their
responses. In two cases where both parents were deceased, the former patient was
taken as the primary respondent.

**Statistical significance of the
cross-tabulations were obtained by the
Chi-Square statistic, at $p < .05$.

by adjustment at the time of follow-up
so as to ascertain how the patient's
functioning years after admission to the
hospital was related to his life before
and during hospitalization. Then, the
selected variables were cross tabulated
by diagnostic category as defined by the
"Discharge Diagnosis" in the hospital
record, to discover the relationship of
the patient's life and functioning before, during and after hospitalization to
the particular diagnostic category describing him psychiatrically. Finally,
the adjustment ratings made on the basis
of time were cross-tabulated to see if
and how these ratings were related to
each other.

Organization of Findings

The wealth of basic data to begin
with, plus the multitude of cross-tabular
analyses, would seem to present an overwhelming complex picture, but the data
showed many consistent patterns, enabling
a description of the patients along meaningful and relevant dimensions from early
childhood to adolescence, from hospitalization to approximately five years later.

This study will begin by describing
the patient's life before hospitalization
(Chapter II), during hospitalization
(Chapter III) and at a point in time several years later (Chapter IV). Chapter V
describes the relationship of the subject's outcome to his life before and during hospitalization, in an effort to
assess what variables are associated with
outcome. Three individual histories are
documented in Chapter VI, and reactions

to the hospitalization experience described in Chapter VII. Chapter VIII,
Perspectives, reviews some of the findings
and their implications. The final chapter, Epilogue, includes an interpretation
of the findings in this study in the light
of a recent follow-up investigation of a
sample of adolescents treated at McLean a
decade later.

REFERENCES

1. Annesley, P. Psychiatric Illness in
    Adolescent Presentation and Prog-
    nosis. J. Ment. Sci. 107:268-278,
    1961.

    Carter, A. The Prognostic Factors of
    Adolescent Psychoses. J. Ment.
    Sci. 88:31-81. 1942.

    Masterson, J. Prognosis in Adoles-
    cent Disorders. Amer. J. Psychiat.
    114:1097-1103, 1958.

    Warren, W. A Study of Adolescent
    Psychiatric Inpatients and the Out-
    come Six or More Years Later: II.
    The Follow-up Study. J. Child
    Psychology & Psychiatry. 6:141-160,
    1965.

2. Beavers, W. and Blumberg, S. A Follow-
    up Study of Adolescents Treated in
    an Inpatient Setting. Dis. Nerv.
    Syst. 29:606-612, 1968.

Garber, B. Follow-up Study of Hospitalized Adolescents. New York,
London: Bruner/Mazel, 1972.

Gossett, J. and Lewis, J. Follow-up
Study of Former Inpatients of the
Adolescent Service, Timberlawn Psychiatric Center. Timberlawn Foun-
dation Report No. 37, 1969.

Hartmann, E., Glasser, B., Greenblatt,
M., Solomon, M.H., and Levinson, D.
J. Adolescents in a Mental Hospi-
tal. New York: Grune and Stratton,
Inc., 1968.

Hartmann, E., Glasser, B., and Herrera,
M.A. Adolescent Inpatients: Five
Years Later. Seminars in Psychi-
atry. 1:66-78, 1969.

King, L. and Pittman, G. A Six Year
Follow-up Study of Sixty-five Adol-
escent Patients: Predictive Value of
Presenting Clinical Picture. Brit.
J. Psychiat. 115:1437-1441, 1969.

Levy, E. Long-term Follow-up of Former
Inpatients at the Children's Hospi-
tal of the Menninger Clinic. Amer.
J. Psychiat. 125:1633-1639, 1969.

Pollack, M., Levenstein, S. & Klein,
D. A Three Year Posthospital
Follow-up of Adolescent and Adult
Schizophrenics. Amer. J. Ortho-
psychiat. 38:94-109, 1968.

3. Gossett, J., Lewis, S., Lewis, J., &
Phillips, V. Follow-up of Adolescents Treated in a Psychiatric

Hospital: A Review of Studies.
Amer. J. Orthopsychiat. 43:602-610,
1973.

CHAPTER   2

THE PATIENT AND HIS FAMILY

The sixty-seven patients were all
single, white, predominantly from Northeastern United States, and, as has already been indicated, from the middle to
upper socio-economic levels of society.
Thirty-three were Protestant, twenty-
four Jewish, seven Catholic, and two
claimed no religious affiliation. Age
ranges were evenly distributed from 13 to
19 with the exception of the 13 year olds,
of whom there were only two. There were
slightly fewer females than males, 31
in comparison to 36. (Patient data are
shown in Table 1).

The patients were "advantaged" in
many ways. Their parents as a group
were highly educated; 86 per cent of the
fathers, and 72 per cent of the mothers
had post high school education. Most
fathers had a high occupational status,
predominantly as executives and professionals. A large majority of the
patients, over two-thirds, were educated
in private schools exclusively, or public and private combinations. Also,
most families were financially able to
provide early private psychiatric treatment when the patient began to encounter
psychological difficulties.

15

However, in many respects, these adolescents had lived a life which, because of its "uniqueness", might be considered problematical. Fathers, because of various business or professional obligations, were frequently absent from the home. Furthermore, patients' families tended to be a highly mobile group, most often related to the geographic changes necessitated by job advancement of aspiring executives or professionals. Almost 50 percent had had more than four residences, and 29 percent had actually had seven or more residences.

As one consequence of the families' mobility, many patients had attended a number of different schools. Almost 75 percent had attended two or more elementary schools, and over 50 percent had attended two or more high schools by the time of admission. Changes in school settings were also related to increasing school difficulties, both academic and behavioral, on the patient's part. These difficulties often were encountered early, for almost one-third before the fourth grade. Almost 20 percent had done poorly academically in elementary school; this rose to 43 percent in high school. Essentially all of the patients who were already in college at the time of admission were doing at best "fairly", if not "poorly". Although I.Q. scores were not available for all of these patients, it was felt that they were unquestionably above average as a group, and not at all realizing their potential. By the time of admission, the school situation had become so intolerable that 70 percent had left. Most had attributed their leaving to

"health" reasons; the rest had either quit
or had been expelled.

Two-thirds of the patients had both of
their natural parents as "focal parents";
the remainder had experienced the loss of
a parent (or parents) by way of divorce
or separation, death, or adoption (see
Table 2). Previous marriages and re-
marriages were common. Qualitatively,
family life was characterized by
some   degree of conflict; this was reported for 70 percent of the families.
However, it was not always possible to
properly assess from the data whether the
conflict was primarily related to the
problems emerging from the mental illness
of the child or to other factors specfi-
cally related to the marriage itself.

With respect to family composition,
over half of the patients came from
relatively large families of three or more
children. Considering the number of large
families and the resultant possibility of
"middle" children, only nine patients were
so placed. On the other hand, 20 were
oldest, 16 were the youngest, and nine
were "only" children. Over one-third of
the patients were separated from their
next older or younger siblings by more
than three and often as many as six years.

The influence of grandparents in the
adolescent's development appeared strong
in 23 instances. Nine families had one
or both grandparents living in the home
at some time, and fourteen adolescents had
histories of being cared for in the home
of the grandparents over extended periods
of their childhood. In addition, 41 per-

cent of the patients were cared for at
least partially during their early years
by "domestics" living in the household.

Apart from the family history, the
patients as a group were of interest in
other ways. Birth defects were reported
for eight. Thirteen were characterized
as having significant feeding problems in
infancy, and 11 as having significant
toilet-training problems. Furthermore,
as many as 28 patients were reported to
have had at least two or more serious illnesses,* and 18 were said to have had one
or more serious accidents.

Social relationships were characterized by at least some, if not considerable,
impoverishment. Although preadmission
data classified only a small group, 20 percent, as completely "socially isolated",
there was evidence that many of the friend-
ships described were of a superficial or
fleeting nature. On the other hand, a
majority of the patients had been dating
at least occasionally prior to admission,
and many were involved to varying degrees
with hobbies, sports and/or social groups.

Psychiatric history was extensive, as
shown in Table 3. All but seven patients
had had at least one previous psychiatric
contact prior to admission. Of these, 70
percent had their first contact after the
onset of adolescence, 14 between the ages
of six and 12, and four before five years
of age. A majority of the patients, 55

---

*Illnesses noted were those consid-
ered serious enough to have been recorded
in the hospital record.

percent, had their first psychiatric contact with a private therapist, and psychotherapy was the major form of treatment.
However, 13 of the patients had had their
first contact in a hospital. Whereas over
50 percent of the adolescents experienced
short-term treatment prior to hospitalization, the remainder were, by contrast,
characterized as having had more extensive
treatment and considerable shifting from
one psychiatric resource to another.

In summary, the patients' histories
indicated that they were a rather elite
group in many ways, being all white,
mainly from the northeast, predominantly
Protestant or Jewish, from above-average
income families and highly educated
parentage, and from relatively large
families, often with three or more children and domestic help. A majority had
been exposed to at least some private
education, a number of different schools,
and a number of family moves. Almost all
patients had some kind of previous psychiatric history before hospitalization,
mostly with a private therapist, but
relatively limited in duration.

Table 1
THE PATIENTS' CHARACTERISTICS

Religion

Protestant	Jewish	Catholic	None	# No Data or Inapplicable
33	24	7	2	1

Health History

	None	One	Two	Three or More	# No Data or Inapplicable
birth defects	56	8	16	12	3
serious illnesses	21	17	1	3	1
serious accidents	45	14	1	3	4

Rate of development

	Fast	Average	Slow	# No Data or Inapplicable
motor	12	31	2	22
verbal	7	25	7	28

Education

Type

	Public	Private	Public & Private	# No Data or Inapplicable
elementary	19	12	27	9
secondary	14	19	21	13

Number

	One	Two	Three or More	# No Data or Inapplicable
elementary	13	24	12	18
secondary	24	19	7	17

Table 1 - (continued)

Education - (cont'd)

	Excellent- Good	Fair	Poor		# No Data or Inapplicable
Performance					
elementary	33	13	11		10
secondary	17	7	18		25

	Before 1	1-4	5-8	9 or over	# No Data or Inapplicable
Grade first difficulty	6	11	16	22	12

	None	Some	Many	# No Data or Inapplicable
Social Relationships				
friends - same sex	2	44	14	7
friends - opposite sex	11	40	9	7
dating	21	28	7	11

Table 2
THE PARENTS' CHARACTERISTICS

Focal Parents	Natural	Adopted	Step and Adopted or Natural	# No Data or Inapplicable
Mothers	46	8	10	3
Fathers	48	8	10	1

Divorces #				# No Data or Inapplicable
Mothers	9 (3 now)	2 (now)	2 (before)	53
Fathers	7 (2 now)	2 (now)	1 (before)	57

Deaths Prior to Discharge	
Mothers	4
Fathers	2

Marital Adjustment	Stable	Conflict (of varying degrees)	# No Data or Inapplicable
Mothers (reported by)	16	37	14
Fathers (reported by)	16	34	17

Education	High School	Jr. College	College G.	Post Grad.	# No Data or Inapplicable
Mothers	13	17	13	4	20
Fathers	7	5	21	19	15

Contact with Patient in Early Years	Regular	Alternating	Infrequent	# No Data or Inapplicable
Mothers	63	1	2	1
Fathers	43	11	5	8

Table 2 - continued

Separations from Patient	None	Short	Few Long	Many Long	# No Data or Inapplicable
Mothers	7	5	43	9	3
Fathers	5	4	44	12	2

Siblings						# No Data or Inapplicable
Number	None 9	One 15	Two 14	Three 8	Four or more 8	13
Order		Youngest 16	Middle 9	Oldest 20		22

	Less than 1 1/2 yrs.	1 1/2 - 3 years	3-4 years	More than 4 yrs.	# No Data or Inapplicable
Yrs. between Patient and next older	6	14	4	8	33
Yrs. between Patient and next younger	4	16	4	8	33

Significant others in the home	None	Relatives	Domestics	Other	# No Data or Inapplicable
Early childhood	11	10	18	5	23
Other	48	1	6	0	12

23

Table 3

PSYCHIATRIC HISTORY DATA

Number of Previous Contacts	None	One	Two	Three or more		# No Data or Inapplicable
	7	21	18	19		2

Age at First Psychiatric Contact	5 yrs or less	6 - 12 yrs.	13 yrs. or over			# No Data or Inapplicable
	4	14	42			7

Setting of First Psychiatric Contact	Private Therapist	Hospital	Outpatient Department	Social Agency		# No Data or Inapplicable
	33	13	5	4		12

Length of Treatment (First contact)	3 months or less	5 - 12 mths	17+ mths.			# No Data or Inapplicable
	33	13	7			14

24

CHAPTER 3

THE HOSPITALIZATION

It is difficult to describe what the
hospitalization experience was really
like for these adolescents. The percents
and numbers of who did what and for how
long seem to tell little of the reality
of what they must have actually experienced. Although most were really very
sick at the time of admission, the impact of riding up the long driveway of
the suburban, exclusive-looking hospital,
and walking into the mammoth yellow brick
administration building, must have been a
perception that only the very sickest or
most unaware would not remember and re-
live for years. And, despite the almost
country club atmosphere of the well-fur-
nished cottages and numerous facilities,
there could be no denying the reality
that they were being admitted to a *mental
hospital.*

For most patients, this was their
first admission. The trauma of arrival
and admission may have been less for the
16 who were transferred from other hospitals. The adolescents were escorted by
their parents, and for the most part,
were admitted voluntarily, rather than
under court order (for less than 5 per-

cent). Diagnostically, 23 were admitted for a variety of personality disorders; 20, psychotic disorder; 12, adolescent adjustment reactions; 7, severe psychoneurotic disorders. The most common behavior problems leading to referral were physical agression, bizarre behavior, depression-withdrawal, and suicide attempts.

Many aspects of the patient's hospital course were examined including length of stay, hall residences, therapy, activities, school, casework for parents, home visits, and medication.

Length of Stay

The median length of stay experienced by our sample was 18 months and ranged from 3 months to 9 years. It must be remembered that all adolescents who experienced less than a 3 month hospital stay were excluded from the sample. The clinical philosophy of that period presumed a greater chance for improvement if the length of stay was sufficient to permit ego rebuilding. There were twice as many adolescents who experienced long-term hospitalization as short-term during the 18 month period in which the sample was drawn, so it was felt that this group would have a more representative hospital experience.

Hall Residences

All patients were placed on adult halls during this period with most patients having more than one hall, since they were usually put on the first hall while admission proceedings were under way. Approximately 55 percent of the

patients were on the first hall less than
five months. One third of the patients had
only one hall, the rest had two or more.
When there were changes from halls, reasons included (1) need for more or less
control (2) administrative purposes and
(3) patient's request.

The nurses and the psychiatric aides
on the hall had the most involvement with
the young patients. Interest on the part
of the nursing staff was high but tended
to be mixed with the intense feeling
stirred up by the adolescents. Although
the hospital was attempting to meet the
demands of the new adolescent population,
the adolescents were essentially on adult
halls with staff geared toward treatment
of adults. Although most of the halls
were "locked," this only meant that the
outer door was locked. While there were
some security screens, it was very easy
for a patient to "escape" from the ward
or from a group while on a trip to town,
etc. The patients returned either on
their own, or accompanied by their families
or friends, or through hospital staff who
located them

Therapy

The policy of the hospital was that
each patient have both a psychiatrist-in-
charge, or administrator (who had responsibility for the management of his daily
life on the hall) and his own "therapist".
In fact, approximately 90 percent of the
sample were assigned a psychotherapist.
The psychotherapists were selected from
all levels of the psychiatric staff including consultants, senior analysts and

the first year residents, with the choice
of therapist at the discretion of the
psychiatrist-in-charge. Often it was felt
that the enthusiasm and interest of the
resident was useful, especially for such
very sick patients. The resident's
therapy was always carefully supervised by
a senior psychiatrist. Of those having
therapy, 75 percent had one psychotherapist, and the rest two or three. A change
in therapist may have been related to a
resident finishing his training and moving out of the city. However, other reasons for change included lack of success
with therapy, or the recommendation that
the patient work with a psychiatrist of
the opposite sex. Once therapy was begun,
it tended to continue, with three-fourths
of the patients having therapy with their
main therapists for more than seven months.

Each adolescent was also seen by the
social worker, most frequently starting at
the time of admission. Once the contact
was made, the patient usually saw the
social worker at irregular intervals, de-
pending upon the need, with most patients
continuing to see the social worker
throughout their hospitalization.

Activities During Hospitalization

Although the treatment program for
adolescents was still in the stage of
development, a number of facilities became available as early as 1960. These
included a girls' club, a jazz band, and
a young adult lounge. Other activities
included sports, fine arts, and hobbies
of varying sorts. A large majority of
the young patients had occupational thera-

py, and approximately half held jobs within the hospital (e.g., receptionist,
painting crew, etc.).

Most patients had social relationships both with the same sex and opposite sex while in the hospital, and more
than half of the patients dated at least
occasionally. However, the extent of
their involvement with other patients was,
for the most part, characterized as moderate . On the other hand, approximately
25 percent had considerable involvement
with other patients, and almost 20 percent
had essentially no contact with others.
Contact with the same sex was almost
twice as frequent as with the opposite
sex and, similarly, contact with peer
figures was just about double that with
older persons. Almost all were involved
in relationships with those on their own
hall, but more than one-half the group
also entered into relationships with
others in other halls. Informal social
activities were preferred to those highly organized.

Contact with the opposite sex was one
of the major problems with which the adolescents confronted the hospital. Because
of administrative reasons and parental
pressure, dating was essentially for-
bidden; yet dating was a natural and
healthy desire for the adolescents, and
the hospital records showed that many did
date despite the hospital regulations.

Since many patients did not have
friends in the vicinity, social contacts
outside the hospital were infrequent. The
large number of social contacts and

activities within the hospital suggest
that the adolescents created for themselves a social community which sustained
their social needs during the treatment
process.

School

     Almost 75 percent of our sample were
engaged in some form of schooling while
hospitalized, the majority at the Arlington School, the high school on the hospital grounds. The school's objectives included providing educational programs
tailored to meet the needs of the individual student, carrying out this education in small classes in a regular high
school environment, and placing students
in appropriate schools and colleges after
discharge. Close communication between
the teaching staff and the hospital's
clinical staff helped to assure an integrated approach to each patient-student
that took into consideration his emotional,
physical and intellectual progress.

     The school attendance and performance
of the sample varied considerably according to the individual patient, though most
were clearly above average in intelligence.

Casework For Parents

     Every attempt was made by the social
work department to involve both mother and
father of the patient in a casework relationship. The extent to which this was
accomplished is demonstrated by the fact
that 91 percent of mothers and 93 percent
of fathers had "regular" contact with the
social worker. For the mother this custom-

arily meant weekly or bi-monthly visits;
this was also true for almost one-half
of the fathers. The rest of the fathers
saw the social worker at less regular intervals, but usually maintained contact
throughout the patient's stay. These
statistics are particularly meaningful in
view of the fact that many of these
families came from out-of-town. The
special focus on parents was important to
the total therapeutic process and reflected the hospital philosophy that the
parent needed emotional support during
the period of the patient's hospitalization, and, also a better understanding
of this parental role. For many parents,
casework did not end with the patient's
discharge from the hospital, but they
continued to keep in contact with their
social worker for varying intervals during the post-hospital adjustment period.

     The parents viewed the hospitaliza-
tion as an extremely traumatic event in
their lives, while admitting its function
of giving protection for the child, a
shift of responsibility from themselves
to the hospital, and, in essence, a feeling of relief that the patient was being
cared for. For most parents (70 percent
of the mothers, 50 percent of the fathers)
the patient's problems, and the resulting
hospitalization, had had a negative effect
on the marriage; approximately one-third
said it had no effect, and a few (four
mothers, seven fathers) said it had actually pulled them closer together. Common
feelings shared by parents included guilt
about their child's problems, anger and
resentment toward the patient, each other,
and, possibly, other aspects of the en-

vironment which they considered to have
contributed to the problem.

Home Visits

During hospitalization, many of the
patients were allowed to make visits home,
ranging from overnight visits to visits of
a month or more. The majority of the
patients were allowed overnight visits
and one to two day visits, and 18 percent were even permitted visits up to a
month or longer. Almost 50 percent of
the patients left the hospital at least
once without permission.

Medication

Although medication was prescribed
for this population ranging from minor to
major tranquilizers, there was no attempt
made in this study to analyze the types
used and their extent. The hospital
atmosphere was generally responsive to
dynamically-oriented and milieu techniques as a method of reaching adolescent
patients, and resorted to medication somewhat reluctantly but out of necessity in
more difficult situations.

Discharge

For many patients, efforts were made
to provide rehabilitative transitional
opportunities before discharge, bridging
the gap between the hospital and the
community, but it was well understood
that the post-hospital adjustment would
be fraught with difficulty. For about
one-fourth of the patients this was made
easier because of the continuity in

therapy with the same psychiatrist and/or
the social worker.

Most of the patients, 43, left the
hospital with the hospital's consent; however, eight left on their own against consent (including four "escapes"), and nine
left because their parents terminated
hospitalization (against the hospital's
consent). At discharge, eight patients
were reported by their administrative doctors to be much or greatly improved; 26
moderately improved; 15 slightly improved;
and seven unchanged.

The largest number, 26, went to their
parental home, 11 to live alone or with
friends, two to live with their spouses.
Twelve were transferred to other hospitals, and a few more to different facilities, including half-way houses and
treatment schools.

Although the experience of these
adolescents can be described globally to
a certain extent, their particular experiences were affected by the type or
degree of their individual pathology.
Individual diagnoses varied from admission to discharge, reflecting not only
shifts in symtomology but also differences among psychiatrists making the
diagnoses. The discharge diagnoses were
considered more reliable because they
were determined on the basis of the
patient's total hospital experience. The
distribution of the varying diagnoses at
discharge remained almost identical to
that at admission, despite changes:
psychotic disorder 24; personality disorder 25; adolescent adjustment reaction

8; and 7 severe psychoneuroses.

Hospitalization Variables as Related to
   Mental Status Ratings

The *mental status* ratings, described in Chapter 1, were made by our raters on the basis of information in the hospital records describing the patients' degree of pathology, first at the time of admission, and then at the time of discharge. These ratings, shown in Table 4, indicate that the proportion of patients rated as GOOD in *mental status* rose from 0 percent at admission to 19 percent at discharge, while the proportion of patients rated as POOR in *mental status* decreased from 29.8 percent at admission to 14.3 percent at discharge. Furthermore, a total of 31.7 percent of the patients had improved in some way (either from POOR to FAIR or FAIR to GOOD); 66.7 percent had stayed the same; and 1.6 percent (1 patient) had worsened. Thus, at discharge, as compared with at admission, there were more patients showing GOOD *mental status,* and fewer patients showing POOR *mental status.* On the other hand, only approximately one-third improved, whereas two-thirds stayed the same.

Chi Square analysis on the relationship between *mental status* ratings at discharge and various aspects of hospitalization showed several statistically significant relationships.

Admission Variables. *Mental status* ratings were not related to referral source (most were referred by a psychiatrist), number of McLean admissions (for

most patients, this was their first admission), or source of payment. However,
mental status was significantly related to
legal status at admission, with patients
with POOR ratings having proportionally
more non-voluntary legal statuses. Patients with POOR *mental status* were significantly more often admitted as a transfer from another hospital, rather than for
acute events precipitating hospitalization.

Referral Behavior. There was a significant relationship between *mental status*
ratings and referral for hallucination,
delusions, and destructive behavior. In
general, patients with POOR *mental status*
ratings had psychotic or affective behavior problems (hallucinations, bizarre
behavior, depression, suicide attempts),
whereas patients with FAIR *mental status*
ratings had acting-out problems such as
stealing, conflict with parents, sexual
activity, and school truancy.

Halls. There was no relationship
between *mental status* and the number of
halls lived in, but there was a significant relationship between *mental status*
and the number of months in the first
hall. Ninety percent of the POOR *mental
status* patients were in their first hall
for less than four months; the extent of
their disturbance necessitated a change
to a hall geared to sicker patients (more
control, special staff, etc.).

Therapy. There was no relationship
between *mental status* and time between
admission and first contact with a social
worker or therapist. Almost all patients
were seen soon after admission, and better

or worse *mental status* did not hasten or
delay contact. *Mental status* was significantly related to the number of therapists, length of therapy, and when therapy
was terminated. Patients with GOOD *mental
status* at discharge had usually had one
therapist, in relatively long-term contact, with the therapy continuing at least
until and, often, after discharge. Patients with POOR *mental status* at discharge more often had had no therapist or
else several therapists, with contact with
the main therapist for a shorter time
(despite longer hospitalization), and with
therapy not even continuing until discharge, much less after discharge.

Involvement in Activities During
Hospitalization. It was surprising to
find that patients with POOR *mental status*
were as involved in hospital activities
and social relationships as were patients
with GOOD or FAIR ratings.

As would be expected, patients with
POOR *mental status* were granted fewer
visits from the hospital. This was true
for both long and short visits, but the
relationship was statistically significant
only for overnight visits.

Condition at Discharge. There was
a significant relationship between *mental
status* ratings and the staff's estimate
of the patient's progess during hospitalization with most of the POOR *mental status*
patients being rated as unimproved. There
was also a significant relationship between
mental status and termination procedure; a
majority of the patients with POOR *mental
status* at discharge were discharged with-

out the consent of the hospital. There
was also a tendency for more of the patients rated as POOR to be discharged to
another hospital, but the relationship
between *mental status* at discharge and
destination after discharge was not a
definitive one.

Hospitalization Variables as Related to
  Diagnosis

     Mental status was not extensively re-
lated to diagnosis, either at admission or
discharge, although there was a tendency
for patients diagnosed as psychotic to have
a *mental status* rating of POOR. Table 5
shows that patients diagnosed as psychotic
had been more often referred for bizarre,
depressive and hallucinating behavior, and
they frequently had long hospitalizations.
They also frequently terminated against
the hospital's consent, and the staff's
estimate of progress was "unimproved" for
almost 60 percent. Those diagnosed as
having psychoneurotic or personality disorders were usually rated as "improved" at
discharge. Neurotic patients had a shorter
length of hospitalization and tended to be
less involved in organized hospital activities. The patients diagnosed as personality disorders, while rated as improved,
did poorly in school while in the hospital
and ended therapy before discharge. The
patients with adjustment reactions had a
shorter hospitalization (like the psychoneurotic group), but frequently terminated
against the hospital's consent (like the
psychotic group).

     Thus, referral behavior, length of
hospitalization, the staff's prognosis,

and whether the patient was discharged
with or against hospital consent, differed
somewhat according to the patient's diagnosis. Patients diagnosed as psychotic
had a greater likelihood of having a
mental status rating of POOR at discharge,
and thus we see POOR *mental status* associated with these same variables.

   In summary, almost all the adolescents
were hospitalized voluntarily, and were
seen by both a social worker and therapist,
with contact usually at least several times
per week. Milieu therapy included a number
of activities revolving around work, school
and social groups. Many patients made
friends in the hospital, and the less sick
patients were allowed visits away from
the hospital.

   Most parents were seen by a social
worker on a regular basis during the
course of their child's hospitalization,
and expressed a strong need for this
support. Many of the parents blamed themselves (as well as the patient and the environment) for their child's problem, and
at least half said the problems had had a
negative effect on their marriage. None-
theless, most parents were thankful for the
relief and protection which hospitalization afforded.

   The average length of hospital stay
was 18 months, and most patients were discharged to their own or parental homes.
The rest were transferred to another hospital or treatment facility, with a few
going directly to live at school or with
friends.

    Patients with POOR   *mental status*
at discharge were more likely to have been
hospitalized on court order, to have been
admitted as a transfer from another hospital, to have displayed psychotic or affective behavior problems (rather than acting-
out problems), to have had either no therapist or several therapists for a short
time, to have terminated therapy before
discharge, to have been granted fewer
visits from the hospital, to have been
rated unimproved at discharge, to have
been discharged without the consent of the
hospital, and to have been diagnosed as
psychotic. Conversely, patients with GOOD
mental status at discharge more often had
been hospitalized for acting-out, person-
ality-disorder problems, had continued
with one therapist until and sometimes
after discharge, and had been involved in
hospital activities and social relationships while hospitalized.

TABLE   4

MENTAL STATUS RATINGS AT ADMISSION   AND DISCHARGE

	Admission	Discharge
GOOD	0 (0%)	12 (19.0%)
FAIR	47 (70.1%)	42 (66.7%)
POOR	20 (29.8%)	9 (14.3%)

CHANGES IN MENTAL STATUS RATINGS BY PATIENT

IMPROVED

Fair to Good	9
Poor to Good	3
Poor to Fair	8
	20

SAME

Fair	34
Poor	8
	42

WORSE

Fair to Poor	1

TABLE 5

HOSPITAL VARIABLES RELATED TO
DISCHARGE OR ADMISSION DIAGNOSIS

Psychotic Disorders

Referral behavior - bizarre behavior, depression, hallucination

Longer hospitalization

No social relations in hospital

Terminated against advice

Estimate of progress: Improved least

Personality Disorders

Poor performance in hospital schooling

Short time on first hall

Therapy ended before discharge

Estimate of progress: Improved

Psychoneurotic Disorders

Shorter hospitalization

No involvement in fine arts or organized social groups in hospital

Progress: Improved

Estimate of Progress: Improved

Adolescent Adjustment Reaction

Referral behavior: aggression

Short length of hospitalization

Terminated against advice

41

CHAPTER 4

THE PATIENT AT FOLLOW-UP*

What has happened to the 67 former patients, now to be referred to as "subjects"? Did those who had improved during hospitalization continue to improve, or were the effects of treatment short-lived? Did they obtain further treatment in other facilities? What were they like as young adults, having gone through the period of adolescence, a psychiatric hospitalization, and then several years of later teens or early twenties? Had they been able to go to school or work? Had they been able to leave their parents and begin lives of their own? Were they in any sense living as "normal" young adults?

The follow-up data, analyzed from the primary respondents,** interviews (47

---

*Some of the data in this chapter were presented in a paper: From Psychiatric Hospital to Community: What Happens to the Adolescent Patient, (Grob, M., Edinburg, G., Stanton, A., and Mintz, N.) at the January, 1970 annual meeting of the American Orthopsychiatric Association.

**Where more than one interview was obtained from the patient and his family, the correlation between responses from the different family members was extremely high, averaging over r = .90.

mothers, 15 fathers, and 2 patients), indicated that most subjects were in close
contact with their families. Although
almost all of them were no longer living
with their families, the families were
very aware of where the subject was, and
how he was doing. Most families were
very pleased with how their child had done
since hospitalization. When asked to compare the subjects' current status with
that at the time of admission to the hospital, the parents indicated a general improvement for 87.5 percent,* an improved
relationship with Mother, for 67.3 percent,
and an improved relationship with Father
for 70.4 percent. These data were substantially confirmed in the clinical ratings of the subjects' adjustment made on
the basis of the follow-up interviews
(Table 6). Approximately two thirds of
the subjects were rated as having GOOD
adjustment with respect to *mental status,
relationship with Mother and relationship with
Father*. Almost no subjects had POOR ratings on adjustment to *Mother* or to *Father*,
but twenty percent had POOR *mental status* .
The areas where subjects had done less
well were *relationship to peers* (27.8 percent POOR) and *work/school adjustment* (21.4
percent POOR).

Although there was a trend for sustained improvement with maturation, there
were some whose sustained level was poor.
This was supported by the finding of no
relationship between age and functioning
at follow-up.

---

*See footnote on Table 6.

Personal and Family Data

     Of the original group of 67, 6 were
now deceased: 4 were suicides, 1 was
listed as a victim of a homicide, and 1
was reported to be the result of a cere-
bral hemorrhage which occured in a psychiatric hospital abroad. Three of the suicides had taken place during a later hospitalization experience, and the fourth,
several months after the subject's discharge. The youngest subject was now 19
years old; the oldest, 28.

     Some major family crises were revealed
by the data: there were three instances of
divorce between parents (all three families
were remarkably disintegrated at the time
of the adolescent's hospitalization), one
remarriage, and four parental deaths (one
a suicide). There had been some moving
about on the part of the parents, usually
in connection with job changes. In spite
of this mobility on the part of the parents, somewhat, and on the part of the subjects, in particular (as will be shown
later), the families as a group at follow-
up were very closely allied. With few
exceptions, the relationship of the subject with his parents had remained one of
mutual involvement, ambivalent at times,
disrupted at other times, but remarkably
continuous and interwoven. An important
factor reported in the maintenance of the
tie between parents and children was the
separation of residence mutually agreed to
as a means of reducing friction and pressure.

Treatment

Almost all subjects had received some
kind of treatment since discharge, as shown
in Table 7; all but five subjects had at
least one form of treatment, with the settings ranging from public mental hospitals
to private therapists. At least 65 percent of the subjects began their first
treatment immediately following discharge-
half of these at another hospital, and
half by continuing therapy. Forty percent
of the sample had not returned to any
hospital since discharge. Of the thirty-
five subjects who had been hospitalized,
14 had spent less than 6 months cumula-
tively in a hospital since discharge.
The majority of the subjects (44) had received private psychotherapy since discharge.

Subjects with POOR *mental status* at the
time of follow-up interview tended to have
had a greater number of psychiatric contacts since discharge, to have had their
first setting in a hospital, to have had
their first contact within six months after
discharge from McLean, to have gone to
several hospitals, and to have had more
cumulative time spent in hospitals since
discharge from McLean in contrast to the
subjects rated as GOOD, who had often remained "out" for a while before returning
to treatment, and then more often obtained
treatment in a facility other than a mental
hospital.

Similarly, subjects who had been diagnosed as psychotic tended to have had more
psychiatric contacts since discharge, more
often in a hospital, and with more cumu-

lative hospital residence. Subjects who
had been diagnosed as adolescent adjustment reaction had also had many psychiatric contacts since discharge, but not in
a hospital. Those diagnosed as psychoneurotic or personality disorders also had
usually obtained treatment in non-hospital
facilities. Furthermore, subjects diagnosed as psychoneurotic tended to have had
several different therapists and more
cumulative time in therapy than those with
other diagnoses.

Residences

This group of adolescents was as
mobile after discharge as they had been
before hospitalization. Over half of the
group had had more than four residences
since discharge, and twenty-one had actually lived in eight or more different
places. The frequent moves were due to a
variety of causes. Some were directly
related to their treatment (going to or
leaving a hospital or treatment center) and
some more probably related to changes usual
for a young adult (moving away from home,
marriage, etc.). Table 8 shows the trend
of residences from the first residence after discharge (many returned to parents
after hospitalization and many went to
another treatment facility); to the next
residence (many left their parents - some
to live alone, some to live with spouse,
and some to return to a hospital); to their
most recent residence, where fewer were in
the hospital, and most lived alone or with
spouses. Thus, many of the moves can be
seen as directly related to maturation or
to treatment.

The residential pattern for many of
these young people was marked not only by
changes or shifts in direction, but by
frequency of moves and a variety of room-
mates. Their lives after discharge were
replete with brief and, often, abortive
attempts at household arrangements of
varying kinds, including halfway houses
or foster homes, apartments with room-
mates, or apartments alone. Although at
follow-up, relatively few were actually
living with parents, returns to the parental home had been intermittent over the
years, usually for short periods of time,
and most often related to crisis situations. Some had travelled to other parts
of the country, or abroad, but a relatively small proportion at follow-up were
living at a considerable distance from
their home base. This included the few
who clung to the Boston area after McLean
hospitalization even though their families
were from out of town. With this exception, the greater number of our sample
were residing within easy geographical
proximity to their family homes, but
in separate households.

At the time of the follow-up interview, only 7 former patients were still
living at home with parents, including two
in special school programs. Most subjects were living apart from their parental families. Married subjects had their
own apartments, and a few had small homes;
13 of the subjects were living in apartments by themselves, a few others lived
with friends or room-mates. The remainder were in institutional settings
including school dormitories (3), hospitals (7), foster homes (2); and one, in

jail. One young woman was in the process
of migrating to California with a hippie
group after living with them on a small
farm in Rhode Island for a year.

For significantly more of the POOR
mental status subjects, a hospital was their
first residence after discharge. There
was also a significant relationship between *mental status* and living arrangement
at the time of the follow-up interview,
with most of the GOOD *mental status* subjects living either alone or with a spouse
and a majority of the subjects rated as
FAIR or POOR residing in some type of
treatment setting. Furthermore, there was
a significant relationship between *mental*
status and the length of time in current
living arrangement, with subjects rated
as GOOD having lived there for a longer
time.

Subjects who had been diagnosed as
psychotic were more apt to have had both
their first and most recent living
arrangements in a hospital than subjects
in the other diagnostic categories, more
of whom had had their first living
arrangements at home. Those diagnosed as
psychoneurotic also tended to have had
their most recent living arrangements at
home, whereas those who had been diagnosed with personality disorders were more
apt to be living with a spouse. Subjects
diagnosed as psychoneurotic had had, as
a group, the fewest number of living
arrangements; because they stayed with
their parents, they moved around less.

Marital Status

Of the 64 former patients for whom
follow-up interviews were obtained, eigh-
teen had married since discharge, and 12
of the 18 were still married to these
spouses. Of the 6 divorced, 3 remarried.
However, one of these had divorced again,
yielding a total of 4 with divorce marital
status at the time of the interview.

In 7 instances, parents approved of
the spouse and felt the marriage was pro-
moting growth for the patient. It is perhaps more interesting that the informants
felt the marriage was inhibiting growth in
only two instances. Half of the marriages
were rated as "good".

Of the 18 marriages, 10 had no children as of the time of the interview; of
the 8 subjects who did have children, 6
had one child; 2 had two children. With
respect to the female subjects with histories of sexual acting out behavior, it
was interesting to note that the parents
were surprised and pleased at their daughter's total involvement in the mothering
process.

Of those married, none were rated
POOR in   *mental status*. Furthermore, there
was a significant relationship between
mental status   and the informant's rating of
the marriage having a positive effect on
the subject for those who were married.
Diagnostically, divorce was more common
for those with personality disorders, and
marriage more often was seen as having a
negative effect for those so diagnosed.

Education

Twenty-four subjects made no attempt
to further their education after discharge.
Of the 33 subjects who had received additional schooling, 2 were still attending
high school and 14 had graduated; of the
14, it is remarkable that 11 had done well.
Thirty-one of the group had participated
in post-high school education, the majority in a four-year college program. Of
those with higher education whose performance was rated, approximately half had
done well.

Commitments to school programs had
not followed any conventional pattern.
They were characterized more commonly by
changes from one school to another, shifts
in curriculum, and reduction of program requirements. Many dropped out of the educational scene for periods of time, to
return at a later date. Those who were
currently involved in school programs
appeared to be rather well motivated, or
persistent, in contrast with their histories of educational disappointments.
For these individuals, the level of current performance appeared to be higher
than that at the time of hospitalization.
Thus, although a large number had not gone
to school at all since discharge, an almost equal number had not only continued
their education but were also doing relatively well.

There was a tendency for those subjects rated as FAIR or POOR not to have
had schooling after discharge. However,
significantly more subjects rated as GOOD
or FAIR had some type of post-high school

education. Diagostically, those diagnosed as psychoneurotic or adolescent adjustment reaction had the most schooling
after discharge, with those in the psychoneurotic classification having had the
most post-high school education. Although
subjects who had been diagnosed as psychotic had had, as a group, the most
schooling before discharge, they tended
not to continue school afterwards.

Work History

     Approximately half of the sample had
worked at some time, either part or full
time, after discharge. For those who had
been employed, their performance varied
from good, fair, and poor with approximately the same number in each group.
One third of those who had worked had
been employed in at least three different
jobs, with most averaging less than six
months on a job. However, of those
currently employed, over half had been
there over six months, and only 2 were
doing poorly. Almost all of the subjects working were rated as "improved" in
this area, and most were said to have good
job performance.

     The job histories of the former pa-
tients since their discharge were usually
somewhat erratic with considerable mobility over the years in semi-skilled or
un-skilled positions. The trend appeared
upward, however, in the kinds of jobs
they had at the time of follow-up including clerk, salesperson, draftsman,
film editor, buyer, lab technician, and
musician. Perhaps of more moment, they
seemed to be staying at one position for

longer periods of time and described
themselves as having some job satis-
factions. Support of families was evidenced here by way of frequent intervention in providing help with obtaining
jobs. There was also indication that
such intervention was provided for the
husbands of former female patients when
they were not vocationally trained or
highly skilled.

Thus, although work history had not
been particularly good for the group as
a whole since discharge, those who were
working at the time of the interview
appeared to be making progress. There
was a significant relationship between
mental status and work history, with more
than 50 percent of the subjects rated
POOR having no work history. Almost all
of the subjects rated GOOD had a good to
fair work history. Of those who were
working, there was a significant relationship between performance at work and
 mental status, with most of the subjects
rated GOOD on *mental status* doing well on
the job. Of the subjects rated FAIR or
POOR, most were having problems on the
job.

More of the subjects who had been
diagnosed as psychotic had no employment.
Subjects in the personality disorder
category had experienced more work history,
more months at their current jobs, tended
to do well at work and to be rated as
much improved in this area over the last
few years. Among the psychoneurotic and
adolescent reaction diagnoses, those who
worked, were doing well.

Social Activities

About one-fourth of these young people were still relatively isolated socially.
Particularly, there was evidence that among
the unmarried former patients there were a
good number of "loners". Dating was spas-
modic or nonexistent for them. However,
almost half of the subjects did date, and
more than half had friends of one or both
sexes. Three were openly homosexual.
Even for those with social relationships,
there was considerable evidence of frustration in this area. Some tended to have
dyadic associations as a social pattern,
others to move in groups in which they did
not feel close to anyone.

For many, the transition from McLean
to the community had been especially difficult in the social aspects; hospitalization
had left them feeling cut off from their
community ties. Many tended therefore, to
cling to McLean associations long after discharge from the hospital. A very small
number still maintained this contact over
the years and found it meaningful.

Involvement in social activities is
described in Table 9. Memberships in clubs,
organizations and church groups were rare.
There was some participation in sports, but
much less than in earlier years. About one-
fourth were involved in art activities and
half were reported to be regularly enjoying
and listening to music, and/or playing an
instrument, this being by far the most pop-
ular interest. Other hobbies include
reading, collecting items of various kinds,
such as guns or trains, skydiving, writing
poetry, and so on, although the percentage

of subjects involved in these activities
was small. Some of the group were depicted
as having "no interests at all".
Neither *mental status* nor diagnosis were
related to the subject's involvement in
activities, but both were related to
social-life variables. Subjects rated
POOR in *mental status* tended not to date
nor to have friends in contrast to most of
the subjects rated GOOD who usually had
friends and sometimes dated. Diagnostically, those who dated and had friends
were more often those with adolescent
adjustment reactions and personality disorders; the latter were sometimes even
characterized as dating "excessively".
Social life was one of the main variables
which delineated the diagnostic groupings.

Self Management

     Data describing the degree to which
the subject was managing his life appear
on Table 10. The parents were still
assuming financial responsibility for almost half of the subjects. Although many
(46.8 percent) subjects were managing money well, a large number were not. Thirteen
of the subjects were not managing their own
lives at all, 26 were beginning to, and 20
were doing well. Fewer had attained significant "emotional independence" from
their families although a large number
(47 percent) were beginning to do so.

     Mental status was significantly re-
lated to all of these self-management
variables. Subjects with POOR *mental
status* were essentially dependent on their
parents for financial support; managed
their money very little if at all; managed

their lives in general little, if at all;
and most showed no "emotional independence". At least half of the subjects
rated as GOOD were responsible for themselves financially, managing their money
effectively, managing their lives in general, and had attained at least some level
of "emotional independence". Diagnostically, those in the psychotic category
were having the most problems in these
areas, and those who had been diagnosed as
adolescent adjustment reactions were doing
the best of the diagnostic groups.

Problems Still Current at the Time of
   Follow-up

     Problem areas were documented in the
interviews and ranged from clinical status
to personal and social development. Areas
presented as continuing problems are described in Table 11.

     The clinical history of the subjects
showed a favorable trend in the direction
of a diminution of symptomatology after
discharge. During the period of transition from the hospital to the community,
there appeared to be a perseveration of
symptoms. However, at the time of follow-
up, 43 percent of the former patients were
reported to be free of abnormal behavior
manifestations. For those still encoun-
tering problems, impulsivity, bizarre behavior, and depression were most common.

     Most often, even for former patients
free of abnormal behavior manifestations,
families expressed concern over immaturi-
ties which still characterized the personality such as "I wish he were more re-

sponsible - or more social - ". Thus,
almost all the patients had at least some
problem areas, with the most frequent being
peer relationships.

There was a significant relationship
between *mental status* and the number of
problems present currently, with all the
subjects with POOR *mental status* having
three or more problems currently and most
of the subjects rated GOOD having no problems currently, or at most one or two.
Subjects rated as FAIR had at least some
mention of present problems.

Mental status was also significantly
related to the subjects' problems with
authority figures, parents in general,
mother in particular, and siblings. Also,
subjects with POOR *mental status* tended to
have more problems relating to peers.
Symptoms significantly related to *mental
status* included impulsivity, bizarre behavior and depressed behavior.

The type of problems current at
follow-up was also related to diagnostic
category. Those who had been diagnosed
as psychotic had more problems with peers,
siblings, bizarre behavior, depressed behavior, and asocial behavior; subjects
classified as psychoneurotic also tended
to have problems with peers and some depressed behavior; those with personality
disorders had more problems with authority
figures, lying, and court offenses; subjects with adolescent adjustment reaction
classification tended to have the fewest
problems.

In summary, while the overall course

of post-hospital adjustment during the
intervening years was uneven, major trends
were discernible and in the direction of
improvement. Improvement in overall
functioning was reported by families for
the large majority of subjects with subsequent corroboration by way of the clinical rating. Most improvement was noted in
the areas of family relationships and reduced symptomatology; to a lesser degree,
progress was made with reference to education and work; least improvement was
shown in social relationships. Twelve
(or 20 percent) of the subjects were
classified as marginally adjusted or as
POOR in overall adjustment. POOR *mental
status* would also have been attributed
to at least 5 of the 6 patients who were
deceased.

The subjects were seen as a highly
mobile group with frequent access to
psychiatric facilities, more commonly
hospitalization for the psychotic ex-patients by contrast with private contacts
for ex-patients diagnosed otherwise. For
the most part, the subjects were not living
with their parents at the time of follow-
up, but appeared to still be considerably
dependent on them for emotional, financial,
vocational, and other support. Families
and former patients were surprisingly intact with respect to their ties.

A small number of subjects had
married, none of whom had been rated POOR
in *mental status*. Subjects rated GOOD at
outcome were more commonly continuing with
their schooling, making work progress,
tending to have friends and social activities, and beginning to achieve emotional

independence from their families by
contrast with those evaluated as POOR.
Diagnostically, subjects classified as
psychotic tended at outcome to have had
no post-hospital schooling, little employment, little or no social life, as
well as the least emotional independence.

TABLE 6

RATINGS OF ADJUSTMENT FIVE YEARS LATER

	GOOD	FAIR	POOR
Mental Status	38(63.4%)	10(16.7%)	12(20.0%)
Relationship to Mother	31(62.0%)	16(32.1%)	3(6.0%)
Relationship to Father	33(63.5%)	18(34.6%)	1(1.9%)
Relationship to Peers	22(40.7%)	17(31.5%)	15(27.8%)
Work-School Adjustment	32(57.1%)	12(21.4%)	12(21.4%)

INFORMANTS EVALUATION OF SUBJECT AT FOLLOW-UP AS COMPARED WITH ADMISSION

	IMPROVED	SAME	WORSE
General Condition	49(87.5%)*	3	4
Relationship with Mother	37(67.3%)	13	5
Relationship with Father	38(70.4%)	12	4

*This figure is particularly high because it does not include the 6 deceased patients, and 4 patients whose functioning was too variable to categorize.

TABLE 7

TREATMENT SINCE DISCHARGE

	None	One	Two	Three	Four	Five or More	No Data or Inapplicable
Number of Psychiatric Contacts	5	15	13	10	6	9	26

	None	One	Two	Three or More			No Data or Inapplicable
Number of Hospitals	24	16	8	11			5
Number of Therapists	11	33	10	1			9

	Less than 6 mos.	6 mos. – 2 yrs.	More than 2 yrs.				No Data or Inapplicable
Time Cumulative in Hospitals	14	14	7				5
Time in Therapy	6	15	16				16

	None	6 mos. or less	More than 6 mos.				No Data or Inapplicable
Time Elapsed Between Discharge and First Contact	32	8	4				15

	Private-Non-Inst.	Private Hosp.	Public Mental	Other			No Data or Inapplicable
Setting of First Contact	24	10	5	11			9

Table 8

RESIDENCES SINCE DISCHARGE

Number	1-3	4-7	8 or more
	17	17	21

Setting	Alone	Parents	Spouse	Friends	Half-way	Hospital	Other	No Date or Inapplicable
first	6	26	2	5	4	12	3	7
second	10	9	4	3	2	17	9	10
recent	13	7	13	3	2	7	12	7

Duration	3 mos. or less	4-12 mos.	1-2 yrs.	More than 2 yrs.	No Date or Inapplicable
second	17	10	8	3	26
most recent	12	12	15	5	20

Reason for Change	Routine	Leave Hospital	Go to Hosp.	Go to Own Place	Other	No Date or Inapplicable
second	13	16	6	3	8	18
last prior	21	8	6	4	6	19

Table 9

ACTIVITIES SINCE DISCHARGE

	No Participation	At Least Some
Sports	42	16
Church	47	12
Fine Arts	41	18
Drama	55	4
Music	29	30
Other, assorted	29	29

Table 10

SELF MANAGEMENT AT FOLLOW-UP

	Wholly or Mainly	Partially or Beginning	Not at all
Money	22	9	16
Own Life	20	26	13
Emotional Independence	10	23	16

64

Table 11
INFORMANTS' PRESENTATION
OF PROBLEMS CURRENTLY

Number of Problems	0	1-2	3-5	6-8
	26	12	13	9

Major Problems now with	Number of Patients
Authority Figures	9
Mother in Particular	7
Father in Particular	4
Peers	22
Siblings	3
Sex	3

Symptoms Presently	
Impulsivity	17
Bizarre Behavior	14
Destructive Behavior	7
Depression	14
Suicidal	4

65

CHAPTER 5

FACTORS RELATED TO OUTCOME

Many of the subjects at the time of
follow-up had improved considerably from
the time they were admitted to McLean, and
even more so since their discharge from
McLean. To what extent was this improvement related to specific variables preceding, during, and/or following hospitalization? From an examination of
which preadmission and hospital variables
were significantly related to GOOD or POOR
mental status at follow-up, there emerges a
profile of the subject who was functioning
well versus a profile of the subject who
was functioning poorly.

Profile of "WELL" and "SICK" at
   Follow-up

The "WELL" subject was more
apt to have had siblings not too
distant in age from himself, and
to have had few, if any, extended
separations from the mother or
father as a child. Once hospitalized, he was not apt to have
been diagnosed as psychotic, nor
to have been admitted on a court
referral, or for a suicide
attempt. He did well in
school while hospitalized, was

active in hospital activities, and
continued therapy at least through
discharge. The length of hospitalization was shorter than average, and discharge was with the
hospital's advice. Furthermore,
he was rated as having GOOD *mental status* and GOOD *adjustment to
father* at discharge. After discharge he seldom went to another
hospital, and, in fact, remained
out of the hospital for a while
before returning to treatment,
which was usually in a facility
other than a hospital. He returned to school, including post-
high school education, and not
only worked, but was doing well at
work. He had friends and dated
(if he was not yet married). At
the time of follow-up, he had relatively few symptoms or problems,
and was beginning to attain financial and emotional independence,
and an ability to manage his own
life.

The subject who was still "SICK"
at follow-up (POOR in *mental status,*
and thus usually POOR, or at least
FAIR, in the other areas of adjustment) was more apt to have had
separations or infrequent contact
with both mother and father in
early childhood and conflict with
parents, resulting in a rating of
POOR adjustment to father at the
time of admission. Running away
was a common preadmission problem. Court referral was common,
as was psychotic diagnosis. If he

attended school during hospitalization, he did poorly, and
had few social relations in the
hospital. He was hospitalized
for a longer than average time,
but frequently terminated his
therapy before discharge, which
was often against the hospital's
advice. He was rated POOR in
mental status and *adjustment to father*
at discharge. After discharge,
he usually went to another hospital immediately or soon after,
and spent a lot of time cumula-
tively in hospitals between discharge and follow-up. His most
recent residence was often in a
treatment setting. He had not
married, nor did he date or even
have friends. He often had not
worked, or if he was working, he
was doing poorly on the job. He
still had a significant number of
symptoms and problems, had not
really begun to manage his own
life, and had essentially no financial or emotional independence.

Preadmission and In-Hospital Variables as
   Correlated With Outcome

The specific preadmission and in-
hospital variables significantly related
to each of the outcome indices are shown
in Tables 12 and 13. Since many relationships were tested, some could ob-
viously be significant statistically by
chance. However, variables shown to be
significantly related to two or more
outcome indices may be considered to be
prognostic of outcome.

Relatively few variables emerged that were seen to be significantly related to outcome on two or more measures. While essentially no pre-admission variables were extensively or significantly associated with GOOD outcome, three pre-admission variables showed such a relationship to POOR outcome: 1) having the next younger sibling more than 6 years younger 2) infrequent contact with mother and father (including separations) and 3) running away as a preadmission problem. Five in-hospital variables were related to POOR outcome: 1) referral for suicide attempts 2) poor performance in school while hospitalized 3) few, if any social relationships during hospitalization 4) shorter than average time with main therapist and 5) longer than average hospitalization.

Several other long-term follow-up studies of adolescents made similar attempts to extract variables relevant to outcome. In 1956, Masterson[1] found a number of factors to be related to differential outcome. These included: 1) age on admission, 2) diagnosis, 3) length of hospitalization, 4) length of onset, 5) history of poor pre-morbid social and school adjustment, and 6) prognosis at discharge. Warren[2] in 1965, examining many pre-morbid factors, such as length of onset of illness, physique, socio-economic status, etc. concluded that they had little or no effect on outcome.

Since then, both Hartmann[3] in 1968 and Garber[4] in 1972 have examined their follow-up data for evidence of predictor variables. Hartmann found four demo-

graphic variables significantly related to
outcome: early separation from the father
and early separation from the mother were
found to be related to poor outcome; chumships during adolescence and good object
relations in the past were both related to
a good outcome. In-hospital variables were
considered not to bear any relation to outcome with one exception: discharge to
another hospital was related to a worse
outcome than discharge home or elsewhere.
Psychotherapy after discharge showed some
positive correlations with outcome, whereas variables dealing with psychotherapy in
the hospital were not all related to outcome. A longer length of hospital stay
was somewhat related to negative outcome.

        Garber identified the following hospi-
tal variables as associated with functioning at follow-up: 1) length of stay in the
hospital 2) discharge diagnosis 3) involvement with the adolescent group 4)
medication in the hospital 5) involvement
and interest of the staff and 6) optimism
of the staff. The two best predictors
were medications in the hospital and involvement and interest of the staff.
Those patients who had no medication in
the hospital were functioning on a higher
level at follow-up. This reflected the
hospital's philosophy that medication was
only used as a last resort.

        A review of findings from all these
studies, including ours, suggests that
there are some similarities between them.
For one thing, relatively few of the total
number of variables considered were related to outcome. Three variables did
emerge as common to several studies:

1) early separation from parents, 2) social relationships or chumships, either pre-hospital or during hospitalization, and 3) length of hospital stay.

The (discharge) diagnosis was considered to be a predictor variable in two of the studies mentioned. In our investigation the relationships between the various ratings of adjustment to diagnosis were not statistically significant. However, GOOD *mental status* and GOOD *adjustment to mother, father, peers, and work/school* were most common for subjects who had been diagnosed as adolescent reactions or psychoneurotic disorders. In fact, as shown in Table 14, there was a consistent trend for the percentage of subjects rated as GOOD in each area to be highest in the adolescent reaction category, somewhat less for the neurotic, still less for the personality disorder and least for the psychotic disorders. Furthermore, the relationship of diagnostic category to the subject's life since discharge, (Table 15), shows that those with a diagnosis of psychotic reaction had done least well, and those diagnosed as adolescent reaction had progressed the most, with those in the other two diagnostic categories also doing well in many areas.

Relationship Between Level of Adjustment
    Ratings

Level of adjustment ratings were made on our sample patients at admission, discharge, and outcome on the five dimensions noted: *mental status, adjustment to mother, adjustment to father, adjustment to peers, and work/school,* and the interrelationships of

these various ratings were examined. Data
were not always available for rating all
the dimensions at each of the time intervals sought, but not to the extent that
the comparisons were seriously limited.

In all, 47 patients had been rated
FAIR in *mental status* at admission, and 20
POOR. Of the 47 rated FAIR at admission,
34 were given the same rating at discharge;
9 improved to GOOD, and 1 was changed to
POOR* At follow-up, of the 34 who had
remained the same at discharge, 17, or
one-half, improved to GOOD; 8 stayed the
same; and five worsened. Four were not
given follow-up ratings. Of the nine
who had improved to GOOD at discharge, 8
remained GOOD; one dropped to FAIR. The
one patient who had gone from FAIR to POOR
at discharge remained POOR.

Of the 20 rated POOR at admission, 8
remained POOR at discharge. Of this group,
4 remained POOR at follow-up; two improved
to FAIR, two improved to GOOD. Eleven improved at discharge (8 to FAIR, 3 to GOOD);
of these, all three rated GOOD maintained
that level; five moved from FAIR to GOOD;
one remained FAIR.**

_____

*Three were not given ratings because
of insufficient data in the discharge
summaries. Of these patients, one was
rated FAIR at follow-up, one GOOD, and one
POOR

**Follow-up ratings were not made for
three, including one for whom there was
no discharge rating.

Of the 12 patients rated GOOD at discharge, eleven remained GOOD at follow-up. Of the 9 rated POOR at discharge, five remained POOR at follow-up. Furthermore, none of those who had suicided at follow-up had shown improvement during hospitalization. Of the 20 patients who had improved during hospitalization (from the FAIR and POOR admission groups combined), 16 maintained their GOOD level or improved to GOOD. Of the total group rated as unchanged during the hospitalization, about one-half improved; the rest stayed the same or worsened.

These findings suggest the meaningfulness of improvement during hospitalization as a clue to later outcome. Particularly, the rating of GOOD at discharge appears to have high predictive value. Thus, condition at admission, as defined by *mental status* was not a prognosticator of outcome, but *mental status* at discharge was. It appeared that the hospitalization experience was a moderating variable mediating the relationship between admission status and outcome. Interestingly, although there was a significant relationship between *mental status* at discharge and several hospitalization variables, these variables were not later related to outcome.

What about the adjustment ratings? The one which seemed to have major predictive value was *adjustment to father* at admission. GOOD *adjustment to father* at admission (Table 16) was significantly related to GOOD outcome in three areas: *mental status, adjustment to mother, and adjustment to father*. Of the five measures of adjustment, it was *adjustment to father* which improved the most between admission and discharge.

Although *adjustment to father* was the most predictive of the preadmission and discharge ratings, *mental status* and *adjustment to mother* were the most significant outcome ratings. (These ratings did not vary with the sex of the child). If a subject had GOOD *mental status* and GOOD *adjustment to mother* at follow-up, he was more likely to have had GOOD, or at worst FAIR adjustment in the other three areas. Problems with mother before admission were not related to outcome. Furthermore, *adjustment to mother* did not improve greatly until after discharge. Perhaps, hospitalization readied the patient and/or his mother to be able to improve their relationship; whatever, adjustment in this area did improve greatly after discharge and by follow-up, GOOD *adjustment to mother* was related to GOOD adjustment in all other areas.

Adjustment to mother and *adjustment to father* at outcome were the two areas in which almost no subjects were rated POOR - only 3 to mother and one to father. In fact, our data show that most of those who were not well-adjusted to parents at follow-up (i.e., those who were rated FAIR or POOR in these areas) had problems in all other areas (Table 17). The importance of adjustment to parents has become an important thread throughout our myriad of findings, and has been substantially supported by other studies as well. According to Hartmann, "Among the interrelations considered, it is especially

noteworthy that a rating of POOR on relationship to family was almost always
accompanied by ratings of POOR on the
other measures and with no improvement
since time of admission. This suggests
that for these adolescent patients, the
first steps in recovery may be in the di
rection of improving their relationships
with family and that perhaps a poor relationship with the family actually pre-
vents improvement in other areas". (5)

    Although it is clear that many sub-
jects were considerably improved at the
time of follow-up, it would be misleading
to ignore the fact that a significant number were still very sick, or at least
having serious problems in one or more
areas. At least 20 percent were rated
POOR in *mental status* and/or *adjustment to
peers,* and/or *work/school adjustment.* Out of
the 60 subjects given follow-up ratings,
only 37 had no POOR ratings, as shown be-
low. Twelve had a POOR rating in one area

Number With POOR Ratings at Follow-up

None	1	2	3	4	5	(in all areas)
N=37	12	5	3	2	1	

(the most common area being *adjustment to
peers*) and eleven had POOR ratings in two
or more areas. It is obvious that having
problems in one or two areas did not
necessitate having problems in all areas.
In fact, ten subjects had ratings of POOR
in 2,3, or 4 areas without being POOR in
the other area(s).

A word must be said about the limitations of the methodology. The meaningfulness of our results depends upon the
validity of our ratings of adjustment.
As has been described earlier, unanimity
was accomplished by the three raters for
all the ratings made at the time of admission and discharge, but outcome ratings
were made by the one research social
worker who conducted the follow-up interviews. Although the outcome ratings were
made on the basis of objective research
definitions, characterizing what the subject was doing (e.g., his symptoms, his
performance at work or school, etc.) these
ratings would be considered less firm than
those obtained by multiple raters. However, in view of the particular efforts
taken to achieve objectivity, it was considered unlikely that this difference
would affect the over-all results.

In summary, relatively few pre-admission variables and in-hospital variables were seen to be significantly related to outcome. Conclusions, by necessity must be tentative because of variations between studies with respect to
criteria for outcome, as well as for de-
fining specific variables according to the
particular treatment setting. Consideration must also be given to the possibility
that although few pre-illness and hospital
variables showed significant association
with follow-up functioning in themselves,
a combination of several taken together
might turn out to have predictive value.

An analysis of level of adjustment
ratings at admission, discharge, and
follow-up, highlights an improvement pro-

cess which was merely initiated during hospitalization but continued, though uneven in course, throughout the post-hospital period. Improvement at discharge, as defined by mental status ratings, turned out to be highly predictive of better outcome at follow-up, although many patients who had not experienced improvement also made progress. The relationship to parents at follow-up was highly related to other areas of adjustment at follow-up and was postulated to be a preliminary factor in full recovery. It was suggested that the improvement begun during hospitalization enabled patients and their families to embark on a process which continued long after hospitalization ended.

Two other major factors in the recovery process cannot be minimized; the maturing of the adolescent into adulthood with the subsequent quiescence of many overwhelming drives, and the availability of treatment resources in the post-hospital period.

REFERENCES

1. Masterson, J. Prognosis in Adolescent Disorders. Amer. J. Psychiat. 114:1097-1103, 1958.

2. Warren, W. A Study of Adolescent Psychiatric Inpatients and the Outcome Six or More Years Later: II. The Follow-up Study. J. Child Psychology & Psychiatry. 6:141-160, 1965.

3. Hartmann, E., Glasser, B., Greenblatt, M., Solomon, M.H., and Levin-

son, D.J.   Adolescents in a Mental
Hospital.   New York: Grune and
Stratton, Inc., 1968.

4.   Garber, B.   Follow-up Study of Hospitalized Adolescents.   New York, London: Bruner/Mazel, 1972.

5.   Hartmann, E., Glasser, B., Greenblatt, M., Solomon, M.H., and Levinson, D.J.   Adolescents in a Mental
Hospital.   New York: Grune and
Stratton, Inc., 1968.   p. 149.

Table 12

Variables Related to Outcome Measures: Preadmission Variables

GOOD Mental Status

Next sibling much younger or much older	(-)
Many family moves	(+)
Separations from Mother	(-)
Strict parents	(+)
Running away	(-)
GOOD *adjustment to father at* admission	(+)

GOOD Adjustment to Peers

Next youngest sibling much younger	(-)
Many elementary schools	(-)
Social relations with opposite sex	(+)
Parents "unavailable"	(-)
Early age of 1st psychiatric contact	(-)

GOOD Adjustment to Mother

Next Sibling much younger	(-)
Only child	(-)
Problems with Mother & parental management	(-)
Running away	(-)
GOOD *adjustment to father at* admission	(-)

GOOD Adjustment to Father

Adequate contact with Father in childhood	(+)
No major problems with Father	(+)
Running away	(-)
Fears & Phobias	(-)
GOOD *Adjustment to Father at* admission	(+)

Positive relationship (+)
Negative relationship (-)

Table 12 (Continued)

Preadmission Variables Not Related to Any Outcome Measures

Sex

Religion

Birth place

Performance in school

Grade at first difficulty

Reason for leaving school

Types of schools

Social relations - same sex

Age of friends

Dating pattern

Involvement in sports

Preadmission symptoms

Psychiatric history (age, number,
    type, length, etc.)

Serious illnesses

Serious accidents

Parent's age

Parent's religion

Parent's education

Parent's marital status (at patient's
    birth & at present)

Parent's marital adjustment

Parental deaths

Parent's occupation

Family income

Parent's illnesses and accidents

Number of siblings older, younger,
    same sex, opposite sex, natural,
    adopted, step.

Mother's pregnancy problems

Illness of siblings

Death of siblings

Birth order

Residential history (number, type,
    length)

Relations in the home

Domestics in the home

Who cared for patient in early childhood

Table 13

Variables Related to Outcome Measures: Hospitalization Variables

GOOD Mental Status

Good performance in school while hospitalized	(+)
Discharged against advice	(-)
Continued therapy after discharge	(+)
Court referral	(-)
Longer than average hospitalization	(-)
Referred for physical agression	(-)
More than average contact of father with social worker	(+)
GOOD mental status at discharge	(+)
GOOD adjustment to father at discharge	(+)

GOOD Adjustment to Peers

Hospital schooling	(+)
Good performance in school while hospitalized	(+)
Long time with main therapist	(+)

GOOD Adjustment to Mother

Referral for suicide	(-)
Good performance in school while hospitalized	(+)
Involved in social relations	(+)
Recreational therapy	(+)
Long time with main therapist	(+)

GOOD ADJUSTMENT TO FATHER

Shorter hospitalization	(+)
Social relations with opposite sex	(+)
GOOD mental status at discharge	(+)
GOOD adjustment to father at discharge	(+)

Positive relationship (+)
Negative relationship (-)

Table 13 (Continued)

Hospital Variables Not Related to Any Outcome Measures

Most referral behavior

Referral source or contact

Patient's age

Parent's age

Legal status

Source of hospital payment

Precipitating event or events
leading up to admission

Quantity or quality of family and
friend visits

Area of family residence

Most extra-curricular activities

Frequency or length of social worker
contact

Problems explored with social worker

Attitude of family members toward
social work

Number of therapists

Areas explored with therapist(s)

Number of and length of stay on halls

Hospital termination circumstances
and procedures

Discharge diagnosis

Hall staff estimate of patient's
progress and prognosis

Illnesses or injuries of patient and
family members during hospital stay

Psychiatric contacts of family members

Marital status changes of family members

Table 14

Percent of Subjects with GOOD Adjustment at Follow-up by Diagnostic Rating

	Adolescent Reaction	Psycho Neurotic	Personality Disorder	Psychotic
GOOD *Mental Status*	85.7%	83.3%	69.5%	40.0%
Adjustment to Mother	100.0%	80.0%	60.0%	44.4%
Adjustment to Father	71.4%	100.0%	52.3%	52.9%
Adjustment to Peers	71.4%	66.7%	42.8%	21.0%
Work/School Adjustment	85.7%	66.7%	50.0%	50.0%

Table 15

Diagnostic Category by Life After Discharge

	Adolescent Reaction	Psychoneurotic	Personality Disorders	Psychotic Disorders
Treatment since Discharge	Many psychiatric contacts Contacts in private non-institutions	Contacts in private non-institutions (no hospitalization) Several therapists, and more cumulative time in therapy	Contacts in private, non-institutions	Most psychiatric contacts Contacts in hospitals Longest cumulative hospitalized
Residences since Discharge	First living arrangements: parents	First living arrangement: parents Latest living arrangement: parents (Fewest number of residences)	First living arrangement: parents Latest living arrangement: alone or with spouse	First living arrangement: hospital Latest living arrangement: hospital

Table 15 (Continued)
Diagnostic Category by Life After Discharge

	Adolescent Reaction	Psychoneurotic	Personality Disorders	Psychotic Disorders
School since Discharge	Most schooling	Most post-high schooling	Often school after discharge	No schooling after discharge
Work History since Discharge	If worked, had improved on the job	If worked, doing well	Most working at present Had done well at work Longest time in current job Much improved at work	More had no employment
Social Relationships since Discharge	Have friends Usually date	More "single" Many had no friends	Usually date Have friends More divorces	No friends No dating

Table 15 (Continued)

Diagnostic Category by Life After Discharge

	Adolescent Reaction	Psychoneurotic	Personality Disorders	Psychotic Disorders
General Management at Follow-up	Best at managing money; Best at managing life; Best at emotional independence	No clear trends	No clear trends	More managing money poorly; More managing life poorly; More have no emotional independence
Attitude Toward Hospitalization	Most satisfied with therapist and social worker; Most favorable toward hospital; Most ameliorative positive effect; Least problems now	No clear trends	Least satisfied with therapist and social worker but felt therapy had a positive effect	Most critical of hospital; Least ameliorative effect perceived; Least cure perceived; Most problems now

Table 16

Percent of Subjects with GOOD Adjustment

	Admission	Discharge	Follow-up
GOOD mental adjustment	0.0%	19.0%	63.4%
GOOD adjustment to Mother	14.8%	20.0%	62.0%
GOOD adjustment to Father	8.6%	43.5%	63.5%
GOOD adjustment to peers	17.0%		40.7%
GOOD work/school adjustment	17.9%	65.6%	57.1%

Table 17

Relationship of FAIR-POOR Adjustment to Mother or Father
at Follow-up to Adjustment in Other Areas

Of the 21 with FAIR-POOR adjustment to Father:

15 had FAIR-POOR mental status
15 had FAIR-POOR adjustment to Mother
14 had FAIR-POOR adjustment to peers
14 had FAIR-POOR adjustment in work/school

(Thus, of the 21, 67% were POOR in all other areas).

Of the 19 who had FAIR-POOR adjustment to Mother:

16 had FAIR-POOR mental adjustment
15 had FAIR-POOR adjustment to Father
16 had FAIR-POOR adjustment to peers
14 had FAIR-POOR adjustment to work/school

(Thus, of the 19, over 70% were FAIR-POOR in all
other areas).

89

CHAPTER 6

CLINICAL PROFILES

Results stated statistically are more meaningful when illustrated by individual histories. A closer look at the unique patterns of adaptation to life for each individual provides a better understanding of the change process which has taken place. The following brief histories are presented here to highlight the course of the three young people who were introduced earlier.* They are not necessarily representative of the other patients in the sample, but their different outcomes - GOOD, FAIR, and POOR - include some clinical characteristics of former patients found in each grouping.

KAREN - An Example of "GOOD" Outcome

Karen had been admitted to McLean Hospital after an acute episode of acting out-behavior, following a two year period of increasing difficulty at home and school. Although she had been referred to a psychiatrist for psychotherapy a year

------

*All identifying information has been altered in these histories to preserve the anonymity of the patient and his family.

before admission, she was seen as lacking
in motivation toward understanding herself and not making good use of treatment.

Background Information

Karen's parents, a couple in their
early forties, were born and brought up in
the Midwest. Her father was the youngest
of three brothers. He felt very competitive toward his two older, highly educated,
and very successful brothers and saw very
little of them. On the other hand, her
mother was an only child, quite attached
to her parents and kept in close touch
with them.

While in the Air Force during World
War II, father had married on a furlough,
and Karen had been born while he was over-
seas. He returned home shortly after her
birth. Not long after his military discharge, father re-enlisted. He had en-
joyed the Air Force life and looked forward to the financial security it offered.
Also, it appeared that service life
brought some excitement to an otherwise
dull existence.

Karen's mother described her pregnancy as uneventful and Karen's early
development as normal. She was breast fed
for six months and bladder trained at two
and a half years. No difficulties were
reported for this period - "Everything
seemed to be normal". Unique to this family, however, were the wartime circumstances surrounding the marriage and subsequent pregnancy and birth.

An only child, as she got a little

older, she seemed shy, temperamental, and easily upset. Temper tantrums were a constant problem. When it came time to start school, she did not want to go, and she continued to exhibit tantrums and over-activity through the years. Most of the school reports indicated that she was an intelligent child but very timid and requiring a great deal of attention.

Karen was doing somewhat better in school from ages nine to twelve at which time she lived with her maternal grand- parents. Her father had been transferred to Texas, and chose to have her remain in her school and with her grandparents who had always been in the family household. At age 13, Karen chose to return to her parents and enter high school in Texas.

For those next two years at home, family life had been quite frenetic as Karen had been belligerent and uncommuni- cative. When she was 15 years old, her parents had consulted a psychiatrist, but she had not entered into a therapeutic alliance with him. Her call home from Greenwich Village, after she had been gone a few days, seemed to be a plea for help. At that time she had not completed her junior year in high school.

Hospital Course

At admission (May, 1962), Karen was described in the medical record as an attractive girl who was frightened and suspicious. Initially, she was quite homesick, but agreed to "stick it out at the hospital". Psychological testing

performed at that time revealed an IQ of
110 with a much brighter potential. At a
treatment planning conference held a few
weeks after her admission, her illness
was classified as a personality disorder.
While there was some concern that she
might identify with the adolescents in the
hospital with anti-social problems, it was
recommended that she remain hospitalized
and that psychotherapy and group therapy
be initiated immediately. It was also
felt that her parents could benefit from
regular contacts at the hospital with the
social worker, but because of the long
commuting distance involved for them, it
was agreed that they would be seen approximately bimonthly, and more often if any
crisis arose.

In addition to her therapeutic program, Karen participated in a "young adult" activity group led by a social worker.
This proved to be quite meaningful to her
as the group engaged in such activities
as cookouts, movie trips, and museum trips.
She also became identified with and
attached to the leader.

In September of 1962, Karen began
courses at Arlington School on the hospital grounds to complete her junior year.
Initially, she was quite apprehensive
about resuming school but followed through
and completed her assignments. Several
months after admission, Karen was considered to be making some progress; in
addition she was beginning to show some
identification with her therapist. However, she still had many .problems with
her anger and with accepting adult control.

Over the summer of 1963, Karen
wanted to return to her parents' home,
reluctant to stay in the hospital another
year. However, she agreed to remain, although there had been a major flare-up of
temper outbursts and demands for sleeping
medication to get her through this agitated
period. By September, Karen was ready to
start her senior year at Arlington high
school and was still working on her intra-
psychic problems. Throughout this time,
her parents had seen the social worker on
a regular basis. Although they had some
question about the extended length of
Karen's hospitalization, they felt there
was little alternative and were willing
to continue.

In June 1964, when Karen completed
her senior year of high school, there was
a good deal of discussion as to whether
she would stay in the Boston area or go
home to live with her family. Father had
been transferred to New York state in the
spring. Karen was quite ambivalent, and
her parents were somewhat apprehensive.
After numerous weekends spent at home,
this was resolved, and in September, 1964,
she was discharged from the hospital.
Psychotherapy, as well as family therapy,
had been arranged locally. The final
diagnosis was personality pattern disorder, schizoid personality with hysteri-
cal and depressive features, and Karen was
considered to be "moderately improved".

Follow-up

An attractive-appearing, responsive
young woman, Karen was 21 years old at
follow-up, five years after her admission

to McLean Hospital. She had been out of
the hospital almost three years. She and
her parents responded immediately to the
request for follow-up and were very eager
to participate. Karen was interviewed in
her own home, and her parents in an out-
of-town office made available to the
interviewer.

Two weeks prior to the interview,
Karen had been married to a young man,
John, 25 years of age, who was also eager
to share the follow-up experience. There
was general agreement among all the parti-
cipants as to Karen's well-being at the
time of follow-up and as to the gradual
and steady progress she had made in her
post-hospital adjustment.

At discharge, she had returned to her
parental home to live and had followed
through on the recommendation for weekly
psychotherapy. She has also been able to
obtain employment and was working in a
clerical capacity at a local library,
where she had been employed for over a
year. Her work habits were described as
good, although she remained a little
apprehensive in her relationships with
fellow employees. She met her husband-to-
be, John, shortly after she had started
working here, and they became seriously
interested in each other. He was working
at a bookstore across the street from the
library and, more recently, had begun to
take college courses at night. Shortly
after meeting John, Karen had moved into
her own apartment where she remained until
her recent marriage, when she moved into
John's apartment. A few months previously,
she had terminated therapy because of her

feeling that she could work things out on
her own. She was free of any abnormal behavior manifestations.

The marriage was seen by all infor-
ants as a good one in which both husband
and wife shared an honest relationship
with each other. Karen had discussed her
illness and hospitalization freely with
John, who was understanding and supportive
toward her. Both were making strides in
attaining independence and were self-
supporting. Their attitude toward work
was serious and planful. Karen emphasized
her genuine enthusiasm about homemaking,
particularly cooking, and both she and John
appeared domestic and comfortable in their
cozy apartment.

Karen saw herself as having made
strides in resolving her dependency on her
parents, particularly at the point where
she was able to leave her parental home to
be on her own. Her parents, in turn,
showed a healthy respect for the emotional
gains she had made and for her recent
status as a newly married young woman.
They saw John as a young man who had faced
many problems of his own, making it possible for him to understand what Karen had
been through. They viewed their own role
as one of maintaining interest but not
intruding. Out-patient family therapy had
helped them to achieve increasing insight
as to their own roles in relationship to
Karen.

Karen was limited in her community
participation, but had several personal
interests, including music, art, cooking,
reading and fishing with her husband.

They had a friendly relationship with a
few other couples and attended church
occasionally.

The McLean hospitalization was viewed
positively - in the mother's words, "she
matured ten years worth in two years".
Karen related to the experience mainly in
terms of her relationships there. In
addition to therapy, she saw as "therapeutic" her relationship with her administrator, social worker, one or two aides,
and several patients; "warmth" in the
hospital milieu was seen as a crucial ingredient to her progress, if not "sur-
vival". She also felt the separation from
her parents had helped her to mature and
achieve some perspective. Both Karen and
her mother stressed the increased self-
understanding they had achieved as a result of therapeutic intervention.

Addendum

A year later, Karen's social worker
had a letter from Karen, in which she
wrote that her father had died after a
brief illness. The letter indicated that
Karen felt comfortable that she was handling things well; she was in control of
her own feelings and was able to provide
support for her mother over this trying
period. Her marriage was stable and happy,
and she was continuing to make progress in
all other areas.

Comment

Karen was rated as having "GOOD"
mental status at follow-up; she had been
rated "FAIR" at hospital admission and

"GOOD" at discharge, turning out to be one
of those former patients with excellent
prospects for "GOOD" outcome at follow-
up. The improvement noted in her post-
hospital adjustment appeared to be sustained for the last two years for which we
have information. She had been able to
separate from her parents emotionally and
geographically and to maintain good ties
with them; they, in turn, had encouraged
her attempts at autonomy. Karen had
demonstrated gains in maturity - through
her independent living arrangements, work
accomplishment, ability to be self-
supporting, marriage, and increasing self-
confidence.

JERRY - An Example of "FAIR" Outcome

Jerry had been admitted to McLean
Hospital in an acutely psychotic state,
shortly after entering college, and
immediately following a heterosexual involvement. He had had no previous history
of psychiatric difficulties or treatment.

Background Information

Jerry was the youngest and only male
member of a family with four children. His
parents had a socially prestigious background, although his father, an attorney,
had never had a flourishing practice.
Jerry's father had become quite depressed
when Jerry was six years old, and had required hospitalization and a series of
electric shock treatments. He had also
had another brief hospitalization when
Jerry was 10 but, supposedly, Jerry did
not know of these events. His mother
glossed over them, explaining the father's

absences as business trips. Jerry's
mother had been a beautiful debutante,
and had made what was considered a "suit-
able" marriage, although she had become
increasingly discouraged about her husband's inability to achieve professional
prominence.

Jerry's mother was very vague about
his developmental history; much of his
care as a child had been turned over to
household help. She reported his birth
as normal and that he walked and talked
at a normal age and was toilet trained
without any difficulty. He had entered
nursery school at age three and seemed to
be above average. He attended private
day schools and, as a high school student,
had gone to boarding school. Although the
family had been told he had an above
average IQ, his performance in athletics
was superior to his academic performance.
His failure to be accepted by an Ivy
League school was a great disappointment
to his parents, particularly his father,
who had expected him to attend Harvard
University and follow in his own foot-
steps as a lawyer.

On his own part, Jerry felt guilty
that he had not been able to fulfill his
father's expectations, particularly in
view of the fact that his three sisters
had all attended Ivy League colleges. The
oldest sister was about to be married;
another sister was in graduate school; and
the sister nearest in age to him was still
in college. The family was not especially
close as all the children had attended
boarding school and mainly saw each other
summers and holidays.

Jerry had appeared to be handling the disappointment about college fairly well; over the summer before his freshman year he worked at a day camp at the family summer place in New Hampshire and seemed to be looking forward to his fall plans. His "breakdown" was a complete shock to the family.

Hospital Course

Almost immediately upon hospitalization, Jerry recounted that he had had sexual intercourse for the first time and was quite preoccupied about his relationship with the girl involved. He also felt that now he was "a man" and could do anything he wanted. At other times he would complain that he was hopeless and inadequate and worried about his sexual capacities. He feared that something terrible was going to happen to him as "everyone was against" him, and he heard voices saying he was "no good".

On the hall, Jerry appeared to be quite isolated and was trying to avoid people. He confused the patients with people from his past. He was especially apprehensive about seeing his sisters and had the delusion that he had raped them. He was placed on medication; within a few weeks his psychotic ideas had diminished considerably. He was able to start on the patients' work crew, doing odd jobs around the hospital.

At the initial evaluation conference, Jerry's condition was diagnosed as a schizophrenic reaction, acute paranoid type, and psychotherapy was recommended.

Group therapy was also recommended, and medication was to be reduced. Jerry seemed to respond to this regime. Although he seemed somewhat depressed at times, his hypomania and paranoid ideas were in control. Arrangements were made for him to start at a local college in February, 1962, and Jerry was discharged on-visit to live with his family and to begin course work. By June, Jerry claimed he was doing well, and his family affirmed this. He had plans for a summer job, again in the family vacation area. Discharged from the hospital program in June, 1962, Jerry planned also to discontinue the psychotherapy he had maintained three times a week. The admission diagnosis was confirmed, and he was considered to be moderately improved.

During Jerry's hospitalization, his parents had two social workers because of their objection to the first person assigned. They saw the social worker fairly regularly to focus mainly on their concerns about Jerry's hospitalization and their wish for him to return to school. When he was discharged, they did not care to maintain any contact.

In August, 1962, the family telephoned the hospital to request re-admission, as Jerry was "talking incessantly and not making sense". He had been working over the summer, dating a local girl and planning to go back to college. The family had put off notifying anyone of his increasing confusion which had started about a week previously, but they had finally become very concerned, and immediate re-admission was arranged.

As September approached, the parents grew increasingly disillusioned in their hopes to see their son successfully undertake a college program, as well as increasingly angry with the hospital; the hospital felt that this unabated pressure from his parents was a factor in Jerry's recurrent lapses. And, indeed, this pattern was repeated two more times, with readmissions in October, 1964 and in February, 1966, before an alternative plan was accepted by the family and finally adopted. Jerry obtained considerable vocational counseling before he was discharged on-visit status in October, 1966. The total cumulative time in residence for the 4 hospitalizations had been almost three years. Following his third hospital discharge, Jerry's diagnosis was schizophrenic reaction, chronic undifferentiated type, slightly improved.

On leaving, Jerry went to live in a cooperative apartment with three former patients, rather than return home. He was able to obtain employment as a clerk. He still required an extensive program of psychotherapy, group therapy, and day and night care, when needed; his condition was somewhat shaky.

Follow-up

Jerry was close to his 25th birthday when interviewed, seven years after his first admission to McLean Hospital. Although he was still on on-visit status at the hospital, he had been living in the community for almost two years. Jerry responded to the request for an interview with interest and made an early appointment

to be seen. His parents were less
willing; however, the father indicated
that he could not manage any time, and
the mother arranged several appointments
before finally coming in. Both Jerry
and his mother preferred to be interviewed
at the hospital rather than in their home
setting.

At follow-up, Jerry made an excellent
appearance and spoke with composure, but
considerable feeling. He had been living
in the same cooperative apartment with
several former patients since leaving the
hospital. He was very satisfied with this
living arrangement because of the sense of
security it gave him. He did not feel
ready to live on his own but made occasional weekend visits to his family. He
had been working for an engineering firm
for one and a half years, having advanced
from a position as clerk to a managerial
capacity. He had also received several
raises. The strides he had made in his
employment situation and in being able to
live away from home, had given him a
sense of independence and increasing
assuredness about himself. Although he
had one or two male friends with whom he
shared some companionship, he was still
not comfortable about dating because of
what he described as "a loss of self
esteem" as a result of his illness. His
main contact with women was in groups or
an occasional party. He participated
occasionally and seasonally in a few
sports but was not at all involved in
community organizations.

Although he was still actively engaged in a treatment program (weekly

psychotherapy and medication as needed),
Jerry felt better than at any other time
since the onset of his illness. However,
he still had to cope with "feelings of
defeat and failure - these feelings build
up slowly and take over". He was aware
that he had not resolved some of his dependency problems - his reliance on his
parents for financial and other assistance,
the need to live within a semi-protected
setting rather than on his own, and the
continued use of therapeutic resources.
He retained an on-visit status at the
hospital in order to be able to return
overnight or for a few days during times
of stress. This had occurred on two
occasions, and he had been able to return
quickly to the community.

His mother, on her own part, felt
that Jerry was not autonomous enough, that
he still needed considerable support from
a variety of sources. Jerry's father had
particularly found Jerry's illness to be
an emotional and financial drain.

Jerry's reaction to the hospital experience was generally positive because
"most of the people cared and this really
made a difference. Being mentally ill,
it's hard to see that they care, now I
can see it - it's been worth it, regard-
less of all the pain, it's been worth it".
He was optimistic that he would continue
to stabilize his adjustment.

Jerry's mother has mixed feelings
about the hospitalization; it had not resulted in full recovery, was too lengthy
and very costly, but she felt that Jerry
had made progress and that many staff

members had been helpful.

Addendum

Two years after the follow-up interview, Jerry was discharged outright from on-visit status, and was described as much improved. He had continued to make progress; his symptoms were under control. He was living in his own apartment and developing increasing confidence in his work and social roles. A year after discharge, he was reported to have married and to be taking educational courses at night.

Comment

At follow-up, Jerry was rated "FAIR" in *mental status*. Although he had made gains in some areas, he still needed considerable support, including occasional day or night care at the hospital. He had been rated "POOR" at the initial admission and "FAIR" at discharge. There was conflict in the relationship with his parents, particularly father, to a large extent because of their difficulties in accepting his limitations and the dependency imposed by his illness. Despite some expressed resentment about this, Jerry's family had maintained their involvement and continued to provide both emotional and financial support, but they were impatient to have him become fully independent.

It is gratifying that the gains Jerry was beginning to make at the time of follow-up were further solidified, as indicated later in the hospital record. Because of the seriousness of his diagnosis

and past history, he will probably continue to avail himself of medical supervision as needed, but the last few years
have demonstrated his capacity for re-
constitution after so stormy a period of
recurrent illness.

JOAN - An Example of "POOR" Outcome

A transfer from another private
psychiatric hospital, Joan had not made
any progress in the year she had been
there. Her tendency to run away from the
hospital and to get into serious difficulties had not been intercepted; in
addition, no one had been able to reach
her and provide any kind of therapeutic
intervention.

Background Information

Joan and her twin brother had been
adopted at two months of age by a child-
less couple who had been married for a
number of years and had longed for a
family. Her father was the oldest of
four brothers, born and brought up in
moderate circumstances. The paternal
grandfather had been a salesman who had
done relatively well. The father was
quite attached to his own mother and the
rest of his family, and took several of
them into his business. Joan's mother was
an only child whose parents had died
when she was very young.

Having achieved a top executive position in a large oil company, the father
traveled extensively and was frequently
away from home. The mother, on her part,

did not like to travel and devoted herself
to raising the twins. The father became
increasingly disappointed in what he considered mother's narrowing view of the
world and her life, as she became more
homebound and involved with the children.

While there is little in the record
telling about Joan's early behavior, the
record does state that she was a bright
child but sullen and uncommunicative. She
was quite competitive with her brother and
often worried about who her "real" parents were. She questioned her legitimacy
and the whereabouts of her biological
mother.

When the children were twelve years
of age, the father sued for divorce. Because he was persistent in wanting his
son, and mother had concern over a financial settlement, it was finally arranged
that Joan would live with the mother while
twin brother, Paul, would go to live with
his father. Shortly after the divorce,
the father remarried, and both children
traveled back and forth between the two
homesteads.

It was soon after Joan's father had
left home that her sexual promiscuity began, and her mother was unable to control
her comings and going. Her mother was
especially horrified that Joan would
flaunt her relationships with blacks or
with people of lower socio-economic background. In addition, Joan's drinking
bouts increased and suicidal wishes over-
whelmed her. In actuality, she never
attempted suicide but had frequent periods
of depression. It was after the second

pregnancy scare when Joan turned herself
into a venereal disease clinic in New
York, that the family made arrangements
for her first admission to a private
psychiatric hospital. Joan had not completed one year of high school.

Hospital Course

The McLean Hospital record described
Joan, at transfer, as rather conspicuous
in her appearance. She was extremely
heavy and had brightly tinted hair. She
bragged about her drinking bouts, her
sexual behavior and ways that she had
burned and scarred herself in the past.
She engaged in inappropriate sexual behavior on the ward with other young patients, both boys and girls, and seemed
sexually exhibitionistic. Her initial
diagnosis was schizophrenic reaction,
chronic undifferentiated type.

She was quickly assigned to an experienced psychotherapist with whom she
worked for several months; he terminated
because he felt that Joan was not bene-
fiting from the therapy and had made little
progress. Joan continued to have temper
tantrums, burst out with obscenities, frequently stayed in bed, and would not change
her clothes. While there were brief periods when she would seem to respond a
little, her hospital course was stormy.
She would leave the hospital frequently
without permission, and she usually ended
up drinking, taking drugs, or having some
casual sexual experience.

After therapy terminated, and until
a female therapist was selected, Joan

appeared quite regressed in that she was
sleeping all day and refused to go to
school a good part of the time. At times
she became suicidal and on one occasion
seriously cut her right wrist. She seemed
unable to make a commitment to the hospital and to her therapy. In July, 1965,
she left the hospital without permission
and went to live with another patient in
a room he had rented. Her discharge
diagnosis was schizophrenic reaction,
chronic undifferentiated, unimproved.

Joan kept in touch with her second
therapist but not on any regular basis.
Apparently, she left Boston and returned
to New York where once again she resumed
her promiscuous, drug-taking life. At one
point she became very depressed and telephoned her father, who arranged for her
readmission to McLean. This was in
November, 1965.

Once more she remained in the hospital for about a year, but again left without permission, this time to live in her
own apartment locally, again keeping in
touch with her therapist. Her brother,
upon returning to the area to attend
Boston College, visited her. He found her
disorganized, dirty, unkempt and, seem-
ingly, in a drug state. He arranged to
have her readmitted in September, 1967.
In a treatment interview conducted at the
hospital at that time, concern was expressed regarding the fact that while she
appeared to regress considerably during
hospitalization, she was also unable to
live in the community in a socially
acceptable way. There did not seem to be
an easy approach to her problem.

Throughout Joan's stay in the
hospital, various efforts were made to
keep both her parents and brother informed
about the problems being encountered.
There were many crises centering around
patient's escapes from the hospital, pregnancy scares, worries about suicide, etc.
The mother attempted to visit fairly regularly but found it increasingly difficult
to offer "support". The father felt
emotionally drained and found it easiest
to separate himself entirely. The twin
brother tried to be a constant constructive
force - participated in joint meetings and
was most cooperative and helpful throughout.

Follow-up

Joan, 21 years old, was interviewed
on her hall at McLean Hospital, several
months after her readmission. It was four
and one half years after her initial admission. In appearance, she was obese and
sloppy, and she avoided looking at the
interviewer directly. She had passively
accepted the request for an interview and
was seen twice because of her limited
attention span and depressed affect. Her
father was not contacted because he had
withdrawn from the treatment program except for his assumption of financial
responsibility; her mother was also interviewed at McLean, after some initial resistance to participating. She explained
her hesitation as discouragement about the
whole process of involvement.

Joan was doing quite poorly at the
time of follow-up. She had been unable to
make any progress in her treatment program

and was very depressed. She was quite
angry about being hospitalized and spent
a good bit of her time sleeping. Efforts
on the part of the staff to engage her in
activities were unsuccessful. Changes in
medication and therapists had not been
helpful. Her only outlets were an
occasional week-end visit to her mother's
home and a relationship with one or two
patients on her hall. Her constant tendency to run away from the hospital and
get into community difficulties had resulted in her being legally committed.

Joan's mother was equally disheart-
ened about how things were going. She was
finding it increasingly difficult to maintain the frequency of contacts. She was
quite critical of her ex-husband's with-
drawal and of the hospital's inability to
affect any improvement in Joan's condition. The only person that the mother
had found to be helpful was the social
worker; "she is the only person I can
turn to".

Addendum

According to the medical record, Joan
had failed to make clinical progress despite the many avenues pursued in her
treatment program. She was able, however,
to complete the requirements for her high
school degree before leaving the hospital
in June, 1968 without permission once
again. The discharge note indicates that
her parents had about given up on her, although her brother was still trying to
stay involved. It was considered doubtful
that she could get along without the strict
surveillance of a hospital setting. Two

months later McLean received a letter from
a state hospital in her home state requesting a medical abstract, as she had
been admitted there. She had been picked
up by the police on a serious legal charge
and was subsequently referred for psychiatric evaluation.

Comments

Joan was evaluated as "POOR" in *mental
status* at follow-up. Her condition was
deteriorating. She had been unable to
engage herself in any aspect of the treatment program. At admission Joan had been
rated as "FAIR"; by the time of discharge
she was considered to have worsened and
was given a rating of "POOR". All efforts
to intercept her self-destructive course
proved fruitless.

Although her mother and her brother
had made considerable efforts to provide
support, her father was alienated by the
continuous onslaught of problems her
illness presented, and the demands on him
which his ex-wife made in this regard, and
he withdrew his contact. Unfortunately,
Joan had been unable to achieve even a
minimal level of adaptation that would
have made it possible for her to remain
out of the hospital.

CHAPTER   7

FAMILY REACTIONS*

The separation of the adolescent
from his family and the community at a
crucial time in his life presents many
problems. Although there are studies
which focus upon families during the
hospitalization experience, little investigation has been done of family attitudes and reactions in the post-hospital
period when the crisis situation is over.
Among our follow-up concerns,we were interested to learn how families perceived
the hospitalization experience in retrospect, and whether positive or negative
reactions were related to subject's outcome. Another area of interest included
parents' feelings toward the subjects at
the time of follow-up, and the relationship of outcome to these findings.

Data for the findings were based on
informant's spontaneous discussion about
the hospital experience, as well as on
structured pre-coded questions regarding

_____

*Some of the data in this chapter
are taken from an article by Grob, M. and
Edinburg,G. How Families View Psychiatric
Hospitalization for their Adolescents;
International Journal of Social Psychiatry,
Volume 18, #1, Spring, 1972.

certain aspects of hospitalization such as
visiting regulations, hospital policies,
management issues, peer relations and role
of personnel. Open-ended questions were
analyzed and classified with respect to
salient issues which had emerged. The aim
was to obtain experiential data as well as
over-all expressions of like and dislike.
This seemed to be a relevant focus because
even respondents who had contrasting feelings about the hospital in general, often
had similar attitudes about particular
issues. It is felt that one incentive for
participation in the study may have been
the opportunity offered respondents to
ventilate their feelings about the hospitalization experience.

As may have been expected, when given
an opportunity to discuss their reactions,
informants frequently reflected on
whether hospitalization could have been
avoided. Some felt that it had been a
mistake despite the apparent urgency at
the time of admission. These feelings
were generally expressed by families of
adolescents with acting-out problems who
now felt the youngster might have been
allowed "to sow his wild oats". The
informants made elaborate references to
the added problems which accrued from
hospitalization, such as exposure to
other sick people, drugs, sex, removal
from the community of normal adolescents,
and that the child had irretrievably lost
an entire stage of his development. "He
lost his adolescence."

Guilt was evidenced even by parents
whose children showed a marked improvement upon discharge from McLean, although

these parents were ultimately able to
justify their decisions in terms of the
resultant progress. These feelings of
guilt were particularly pervasive in
cases where the home situation was something less than ideal. Former patients,
too, tended to place blame primarily upon
the parents. "Leaving home to go into the
hospital at 14 - it's very hard - you
can't help feeling your parent has failed
you", and "somehow if my parents had been
better, I wouldn't have been a nut".
Guilt and blame are thus both experienced
by and attributed to parents.

The problem of guilt was exacerbated
by the social stigma connected with mental
illness and hospitalization. All seemed
to share feelings that the mentally ill
person was "different" and that the larger
community is not usually accepting of him
and his differences. Families tended to
be selective with their relatives and
friends in their acknowledgement of the
illness. There was a general wariness of
the community's reaction. Efforts at
total denial of the illness were particularly conspicuous in the matter of job
finding. A small number referred to the
stigma as a major roadblock to recovery:
a frequent response among those who projected their difficulties onto the attitudes of others and who were generally
alienated from normal society. More significant, however, may be the evidence of
an emerging freedom to share their traumatic experiences with select friends or
family members for relief and support.

There was clearly an element of frustration and confusion on the part of many

parents with respect to their parental
role after the child entered the hospital.
Geographically remote parents, who did not
visit often, showed less concern in this
area and appeared more willing to relin-
quish a major portion of their normal authority. Parents who visited more frequently expressed resentment of the role
to which they felt relegated. While they
did recognize the need to have the hospital serve "in loco parentis", they felt
unnecessarily excluded from meaningful
participation. "You are no longer the
parent when he is in the hospital."
Acting as liaison between family and
hospital, the social work department
served to reduce such feelings, but was
not always sufficient to overcome them.

Some parents also complained about
the unavailability of the medical staff to
them. Many respondents construed a lack
of communication as an absence of appreci-
ation for their concerns as parents, which,
for them, reflected their already diminished status in the eyes of the community.
"We were shut out." - "I had the feeling
they were never quite telling you the whole
truth." - "I felt like a brick-layer", the
last a comment from a father who, himself,
was in the medical profession. There was
repeated reference to the wish for more
information about the illness: "It was
hard to find out what was wrong with my
daughter - they seem to keep you in the
dark"; another, "The whole illness is
mysterious - the diagnosis, prognosis.
The very point of communication becomes
more important from the parent's point of
view." Such feelings were expressed by
many families notwithstanding their re-

porting of favorable outcome. By contrast,
quite often when communication with the
therapist met the parents' needs, their
attitude toward the hospital was positive,
irrespective of favorable or unfavorable
outcome. From a parent who had easy access
to the doctor, "He (the doctor) talked in
terms we could understand. I felt we were
participating more. We could appreciate
all that was going on - we were understanding of treatment." Another parent
described the importance of communication
this way: "We're all better for her illness - have a better understanding of life
and how to cope - we were guilty - we're
better now - the whole experience left
me weak but knowledgeable."

    Other common issues raised by parents
included: (1) the impersonal character of
the institutional setting; (2) the deleter-
ious effect of lengthy hospital stay upon
the reintegration into community life; (3)
undue emphasis on clinical psychiatry as
the therapeutic technique for adolescents
and insufficient attention to after-care
and rehabilitation work; (4) the inherent
conflict between the training and therapeutic functions of the hospital with the
attendant problem of frequently shifting
personnel; (5) the confusion engendered in
adolescent patients by the division of
role between administrator and therapist;
and lastly, (6) the problem of financial
hardship resulting from the high costs of
patient care. All of these issues have
challenged mental health workers in this
decade. Thus, families appeared to be
quite sensitive to the same basic concerns
which continue to plague professionals
in this field.

Over 50 percent of the families had a
negative view of the subjects hospitalization in general, and treatment in particular. These families tended to be mainly
critical with very few positive things to
say. Approximately twenty percent were
generally favorable, and the rest had
mixed reactions. When asked who was most
helpful to them in the hospital, over 25
percent said no-one; however, for the rest
who acknowledged being helped, social
workers were rated as most helpful, ad-
ministrators next, and therapists last.
Specific reactions to therapists, social
workers and nurses are shown in Table 18.
The extent of contact with therapists was
adequate for only one-third of the parents,
with the rest having had no contact at all,
or less than adequate amount of contact.
Contact with social workers was seen as
being the most adequate. On the other
hand, the effect of the therapists per se,
as well as social workers, was seen as
relatively high, with some ambivalent reactions toward the social workers. Included in these mixed responses toward
social workers were the parents who de-
murred at seeing the social worker in
lieu of the doctor. Although criticism
toward hospitalization in general was pervasive, approximately half of the parents
expressed at least some satisfaction with
the staff members themselves, including
the therapist, social worker, and nurse.

Almost one-half of the informants
reported inconsistencies in the hospital
management of the patient, either from
doctor to doctor on the same hall, doctor
to doctor on different halls, or a combination of both. Less than one-half found

management changes in the patient's program helpful. Parents were particularly
upset by hall transfers which were necessitated by changes in the patient's condition. Some were also bothered by lack
of restrictions to the patient, particularly with respect to off-ground privileges, money, drugs and boy-girl relations.

Many parents were also troubled by
the effect of patient-association. Relatively few, 22.6 percent, felt that peer
associations were helpful, whereas the
rest thought their effect was at best
"mixed", if not "troublesome." The effect
of association with older patients was
seen as being more helpful; "mixed" or
"troublesome" for only 15 percent, and
actively helpful for approximately one-
third of the patients.

Virtually all parents felt that the
visiting regulations were fair and adequate. Visiting privileges were quite
broad, but could be restricted according
to the needs of the patient. Families
generally accepted this policy.

Almost 73 percent of the respondents
acknowledged the necessity of the hospital's assumption of the management of the
patient, although the remainder expressed
some conflict concerning this transfer of
responsibility. Respondents denied being threatened by the role of the hospital
"in loco parentis" in relinquishing their
parental authority; if anything, they
seemed relieved. Apparently their general
frustration related to other parental
concerns rather than their authority per se.

On the whole, parents did not per-
ceive the hospitalization as resulting in
cure of their child's problems. Only 3
perceived their child as "cured", and only
another 13 perceived a specific therapeutic change; most perceived no change.
On the other hand, most parents did see
the hospitalization serving an ameliorative function - e.g., relieving them of
responsibility and of home tensions, and
protection of the patient and/or society.
Of course, most parents, 63.8 percent,
wished the hospital had been able to
effect more therapeutic changes.

The relationship between the family's
reaction to the subject's hospitalization
and the subject's *mental status* at follow-
up indicated that the subject's *mental
status* was not significantly related to the
informant's estimate of the effects of
contact with nurses, social worker or
therapist or of the effect of therapy per
se. However, there was a statistically
significant relationship between *mental
status* ratings and satisfaction with the
main therapists, with the parents of subjects with POOR *mental status* having significantly less satisfaction than the parents of subjects rated GOOD or FAIR. The
relationship of *mental status* to the parents'general reaction to hospitalization
was not significant, although there was a
tendency for parents of subjects rated as
POOR to be more critical. However, parents of subjects of all three ratings
were generally critical toward the hospitalization.

There was no relationship between the
subjects' *mental status* and the parents'

estimate of hospital's actions regarding
visiting, perception of inconsistency in
hospital management, reaction to management changes, or perception of problems
concerning restrictions. However, parents
of subjects with POOR *mental status* felt
that associations with other patients,
both peer and older, had a negative effect
on the subject more than did parents of
subjects rated GOOD or FAIR.

The parents' view of changes produced by hospitalization through therapy
was significantly related to *mental status,*
with almost all of the subjects with POOR
mental status having no changes, and almost
50 percent of those with GOOD *mental status*
ratings having some change ranging from
"cure" to one or more specific therapeutic change.

Parental attitudes toward the former
patient were also reviewed. The follow-
up interview demonstrated that the ties
between parent and subject were strong.
Most of the parents had been in touch with
the subjects within the last month, and
felt they were well aware of their functioning at the time. One-third of the informants saw the subject at least weekly
and only one-fifth had irregular (or rare)
contact. Included in the latter were five
situations in which subjects were described
as having a superficial or estranged contact with the parent(s). This correlates
with the findings in the previous chapter
that approximately two-thirds of the subjects were seen as having improved relationships with their parents. Although
anxiety about a possible exacerbation of
symptoms was expressed by almost half of

the parents, most were at least moderately optimistic about the child's future.

A fair number of the parents had noted changes in their behavior toward the subject since discharge with respect to discipline, supervision and acceptance as described in Table 19. With respect to discipline, over one-third changed their degree of discipline, mostly in the direction of less rather than more discipline. Approximately two-thirds of the parents had changed the degree of supervision, half more and half less. It was particularly notable that the majority of the mothers and fathers saw themselves as having become more accepting of the subject. The reason given for the changes in discipline, supervision and acceptance was the parent's "own idea" for 53 percent, and the result of professional guidance for 45 percent. It is interesting to note that changes were the parent's "own idea" more frequently for subjects with POOR *mental status* at follow-up, whereas parents of subjects with GOOD *mental status* were more likely to attribute at least part of the reason for their change to professional guidance.

The parent's attitude and behavior toward their child varied extensively with *mental status* ratings of the subjects at follow-up. The frequency of contact was significantly less and the quality of contact significantly poorer between the parents and the subject with POOR *mental status* . There was a significant relationship between *mental status* and the parent's having a positive attitude toward the subject, the parent's anxiety

regarding the subject, and the parent's
hostile attitude toward the subject as
rated by the interviewer. Furthermore,
subjects with POOR *mental status* had a
predominance of parents who felt re-
jected by them, and who felt they were
too dependent.

The parent's behavior in the interview itself was related to the subject's
mental status. Parents of subjects with
POOR *mental status* had a general negative
affect tone, whereas, parents of subjects rated as GOOD expressed a positive
affect tone. The parent's cooperation in
the interview did not vary with *mental
status*, but parents of subjects rated POOR
showed significantly more anxiety during
the interview, and significantly less optimism regarding the patients. Almost
all of the subjects rated as GOOD had -
parents with moderate or high optimism.

In *summary*, at the time of follow-up,
families were still struggling with the
burden of guilt and stigma in the after-
math of the experience. Major areas of
concern for families included the role of
personnel, administration, treatment, and
communication. Most families still felt
that hospitalization had been necessary at
the time and had served the ameliorative
function of relieving the tension at home
and shifting the responsibility to the
hospital. However, criticism of the
hospitalization itself was extensive,
particularly with respect to the lack of
communication between the hospital and
the parents, and to the lack of "cure"
resulting from the long, expensive, and
traumatic stay. Parents of subjects with

POOR *mental status* at follow-up were most
critical of hospitalization in general
and treatment in particular.

TABLE 18

PARENTS' REACTIONS TO HOSPITAL STAFF

Extent of Contact with:	No Contact	Adequate	Less Than Adequate
Therapists	15	20	22
Social Workers	3	38	2
Nurses	30	26	2

Effect of:	Helpful	Mixed	Troublesome
Therapists	31	1	6
Social Workers	33	16	6
Nurses	36	11	

Satisfaction with:	Satisfied	Mixed	Dissatisfied
Therapists	31	12	6
Social Workers	37	17	12
Nurses	36	12	2

127

TABLE 19

PARENTAL CHANGES IN BEHAVIOR TOWARD SUBJECT SINCE DISCHARGE

	No Change	More	Less	Total
Degree of Discipline				
Mothers	28	7	13	48
Fathers	34	4	12	50
Degree of Supervision				
Mothers	20	15	14	49
Fathers	20	18	14	52
Degree of Acceptance				
Mothers	17	35	1	53
Fathers	19	32	2	53

TABLE 19 - continued

Idea for Changes	Own	Professional
Discipline		
Mothers	10	10
Fathers	8	8
Supervision		
Mothers	15	14
Fathers	18	14
Acceptance		
Mothers	20	16
Fathers	19	15
Total Percent		
Mothers	52.9%	47.0%
Fathers	52.9%	43.4%

129

CHAPTER 8

PERSPECTIVES

As each of the preceding chapters have been summarized individually, this chapter will not attempt a general review but instead will consider the major empirical findings and their implications, both for this and other hospitalized adolescent populations. Attention will be given to three findings:

(1) Despite the fact that one-fifth of the patients treated by psychiatric hospitalization during adolescence were the same or worse approximately five years later, the large majority of patients had improved over the years and were evaluated as having good adjustment, particularly with respect to *mental status* and relationship with parents, with gradual gains being noted in other areas.

(2) Despite the fact that relationships between parent and child were seriously troubled at the time of hospital admission (particularly between father and child), relationships were remarkably intact at follow-up and appeared to be a critical factor in the general adjustment level of the former patient.

(3) Despite the fact that families

tended to be generally critical of the hospitalization experience, with particular emphasis on the relative lack of communication between parents and the physician, there was some acknowledgement of the helpfulness of psychiatric treatment in the recovery process.

It would appear that these former patients were functioning better than adolescents in some other studies. They were getting along with their families, achieving a measure of independence geographically and emotionally, developing in the area of inter-personal relationships with friends of the same and opposite sex, and making strides in the educational and occupational sphere. In addition, about half were reportedly free of any abnormal behavior manifestations.

In order for us to achieve some perspective on our findings, further comparison with other findings from recent studies may be useful. The studies appearing in the late 1950's and 1960's, most frequently from adolescent programs with psychodynamic orientation, have conveyed a general impression of pessimistic long-term outcome[1]. A closer examination of results reveals a more optimistic expectation from neurotic patients, character disorders, and acute schizophrenics. Poor outcome was most commonly associated with chronic schizophrenics, organic brain syndrome, and borderline psychotics.

Masterson[2], in perhaps the earliest long-term follow-up study of hospitalized adolescents, reported marked impairment

of functioning at follow-up in the sicker
patients, especially those with a diagnosis of schizophrenia. Improvement seen
at hospital discharge, tended to be maintained, however, in the neurotic patients.
In a later investigation, Warren[3] obtained similarly discouraging results for
psychotic patients six years after discharge, again with a higher level of
improvement for "neurotics" and "conduct
disorders".

The Hartmann monograph,[4] documenting
the findings of an intensive study at the
Massachusetts Mental Health Center (MMHC),
found many of their cohort to be still
seriously handicapped by mental disorder
at the five year follow-up, although a
significant tendency toward improvement
was evidenced. Garber,[5] in the most
recently published follow-up investigation
to date, has made a very comprehensive
attempt to transform clinical data into
operationally useful and measurable factors. Our study, in contrast to the
earlier ones included here, is similar to
both the Hartmann and the Garber studies
in its attempt to de-emphasize diagnostic
classifications and focus more on the
functioning aspects of the adolescent.

The findings from the Garber study
approximate ours more closely, as illustrated in the following excerpt: "The
current functioning of former patients
showed that the majority (high and moderate functioning groups) were getting along
adequately in the community. The high
functioning group was making it in all
areas, while the moderate functioning
group showed certain isolated areas of

functioning. But over-all one can say
that 91 out of 115 patients were making it
in the community. This finding was encouraging and gratifying, especially when
many previous follow-ups were much less
optimistic".(6)

In order to more fully understand the
results of our study, a more detailed
comparison with the Hartmann study is
attempted here. It was felt that a focus
on differences in outcome would help us to
derive meaningful hypotheses. In many
ways both sample populations are comparable. They were all adolescents of
approximately the same age, evenly divided as to sex, hospitalized about the
same time (the early sixties) and treated
in dynamic, psycho-analytically oriented
settings. The study population furthermore, was described as intelligent and
articulate, coming from families whose
socio-economic level was above average.

Important distinctions between the
two groups, however, included the
following: The McLean population was
definitely weighted in favor of Class I
and II(7) by comparison with the MMHC
sample which was half middle or upper-
middle, and half lower classes; McLean's
religious distribution had a small percentage of Catholics compared to MMHC -
10 percent to almost 50 percent; and,
whereas, the MMHC study included all patients admitted consecutively during a
particular period of time, thereby involving patients having both very brief
(one day) and longer periods of hospital
stay (up to two years), McLean excluded
all those patients with less than 90 days

of hospitalization. Therefore, it might
appear that the McLean sample was
"sicker"*, an additional factor in this
consideration being that patients at MMHC
were often "selected as a good teaching
case".(8) However, although very sick
patients had accessibility to McLean,
others not so sick were admitted also and
stayed for long periods because their
families sought treatment early and in-
sisted on the "best", which included not
only symptom relief but ego restructure,
involving lengthy periods of stay. At
MMHC, the impression was that although at
least half seemed to be fairly healthy,
young people suffering from "adolescent
turmoil", perhaps a third or half were
severely sick patients. It may, therefore, not be fair to attempt to assess
the comparative seriousness of illness of
both groups at admission, but rather to
assume that in this respect the adolescents
were more similar than not.

What was different or similar in outcome for the two groups? The mean age of
the MMHC study group at the time of the
five year follow-up was 22.5 years, by
contrast with the McLean group, 23.3 years.
It is highly suggestive from the course
of the post-hospital adjustment as described in both studies that the adaptation
of the former patient to the stresses of
life tended to improve somewhat as he
matured. This would immediately give the
McLean group an advantage of almost one
year.

----

*This is also likely because of the
McLean philosophy of accepting patients re-
gardless of the seriousness of pathology.

A major and striking difference was that in the MMHC study most of those not in a hospital at the time of follow-up were still living at home with their parents, a marked contrast from the McLean group as has been shown. Hartmann describes quite a few of them further as "using their homes as small psychiatric institutions and their family members as caretakers".[9]

Another difference in outcome is in the area of education and work. In the MMHC sample 13 of 55 were involved in post-hospital education, by contrast with 31 of the 64 followed in the McLean sample; and where the jobs held by the former tended to be "almost always menial",[10] the latter group demonstrated an upward trend in the type of jobs obtained and held. Although a mean estimated IQ before admission was not obtained of the McLean sample, it would not appear to be markedly higher from that of the MMHC group, which was 115. Therefore, it is not possible to look for differences in aptitude between them as the underlying reason for the contrast here.

The results in both studies appeared similar in two respects, that the least gain over the years was in social relationships, and the most in family functioning, with the additional gain in the McLean group in *mental status* as well. It has already been pointed out thoughtfully in the Hartmann study that an important factor in improved family relationships was the quieting down of turmoil. An additional explanation offered for the improvement in families was the

observation that the MMHC parents were
adapting to the psychopathology of the
former patients. Although the McLean
parents appeared to have lowered expectations for their children than had they
not experienced mental illness, this more
often related to a shift in educational
or vocational aspirations for him, and/or
acceptance of the fact that maturation,
including financial independence, would
proceed at a slower pace, with occasional
or frequent interruptions. It would
appear that the greater improvement in
mental status of the McLean group is the
distinguishing feature of the two groups,
as improvement in other areas (family,
education, and work, and social) is fairly
similar in its patterning, though propor-
tionately higher for the McLean group.

The role of the family seems to
emerge both in the Hartmann and McLean
studies as a significant ingredient in
the post-hospital adjustment period.
Parents appear to be in the position of
encouraging or perpetuating pathology,
and thus interfering with the child's
possible progress. The contrast in living
arrangements between the MMHC and McLean
study population at the time of follow-up
highlights a major difference in social
class expectations and resources. According to the MMHC study, "In the cases
where the patient and his family had
parted, the parting was rarely smooth or
cordial and recriminations on both sides
were frequent".[11] By contrast, McLean
parents encouraged and often supported
independent living arrangements, thus
allowing some separation from the family,
while at the same time maintaining con-

tinuity of interest in the former patient over the post-hospital years. Interestingly enough, although families
maintained separated domiciles, for the
most part they were living geographically
within close proximity of each other.

Other types of support from parents
made available to the McLean group included help with school planning and job
finding, varying forms of financial
assistance, as well as encouragement in
the use of psychiatric treatment facilities. Although both groups appeared to
have similar experiences with the extent
of rehospitalization, the McLean group is
characterized as having more private
psychotherapy and especially more social
work services in the post-hospital period.
The role played by these families in pro-
moting the utilization of therapeutic
resources for both the adolescent and
themselves is typical of their class as
described by Myers and Bean,[12] who examined in detail the relationships between social classes and the outcome of
psychiatric treatment, as well as their
attitudes toward psychiatry and subsequent
use of outpatient care services. Still
earlier, Hollingshead and Redlich had
stated "Persons in the higher classes
hold more favorable attitudes toward
psychiatrists than those in the lower
classes - the higher the class the more
pronounced the feelings of shame and
guilt - interest in the sick member is
stronger, more realistic, and the negative
emotions are less rampant"[13] than in the
lower classes who exhibit "helplessness,
apathy, and lack of cooperation".[14]
Another interesting sidelight, "Usually

these patients and their families make
more demands of the psychiatrist than
other patients."[15]

The McLean investigation further con-
firms these findings. Certainly there is
evidence to suggest that the families
here looked to psychiatry with hope; however, their very optimism about treatment
laid the basis for subsequent criticism
and disappointment with the inevitably
slow and painful process of recovery. Also, recognition must be made of the inherent frustration for families seeking
treatment at a time when the adolescent
population was relatively new in its size
and growing complexity in the mental
hospital field. It is possible that frustrations with the treatment process encouraged an alignment between former patient and his family in the post-hospital
period, enabling them to experience mutual
support and, possibly, growth. At the
same time, despite the criticism and disappointment expressed toward the hospital,
awareness of the helpfulness of treatment
emerged and was demonstrated in the repeated use of treatment facilities, as the
needs arose.

The importance of the role of family
cannot be underestimated. It is suggested
that this might be acknowledged in still
another way, that families be recognized
as "human resources", even as emphasis is
placed on "community resources" as an important ingredient in the after-care needs
of the hospitalized patient. It is postulated further that former young patients
can effect adaptation in the community
when their limitations are accepted by

parents who provide continuing support
while allowing them to experience some
separation from the family. This is not
to say that family relationships alone are
the determinants of outcome. How else can
the number of failures among equally
caring families be explained? Too many
other factors of importance are at play.
It is felt, however, that the special role
of the family facilitates the process of
recovery, if it embraces the dimensions of
allowing the growing adult to separate, of
being supportive, and of maintaining interest. These special characteristics are
not exclusive of so-called "normal" parents. Our study represented a cross
section of parents with varying degrees
of health and pathology. Yet, on the
whole, they were able to project a level
of management and concern which strength-
ened the normalization process.

What are the implications of these
findings for this and other populations?
For one thing, it is possible to say that
one can venture a note of optimism for ex-
hospital patients in that over the years
the process of adaptation to life is in
the direction of improvement. For a small
number, however, the course is downward
and inevitably, doomed to failure. References in earlier chapters have already
been made to differences distinguishing
those who succeed from those who fail, as
demonstrated in this and other investi-
gations. Characteristic for all, however,
is the considerable number of resources
utilized in the return to normal living,
in the form of "community resources" or
"human resources", preferably both.

The McLean study which highlights not only hospitalization but the role of parents as continuing agents in an on-going process, presumes that this factor of resources has generalizability for all hospitalized adolescents. For those populations deprived of "human resources", the community must provide agents "in loco parentis", for equivalent sustaining support and commitment to mental health.

In any event, although our findings with respect to the intrinsic function of hospitalization are not conclusive because of the lack of a control group, the evidence is strongly suggestive that hospitalization is a significant component in the process of recovery for many. The data available on psychotherapy does not permit an appraisal of efficacy. There is reason, however, to consider the effect of social work services on families who were later able to utilize their abilities so well in the management of their growing children. Surely, if parents play so pivotal a role in the post-hospital experiences of their children, more attention to the understanding of their parental role can serve to enlighten and support them during trying periods.

These adolescents were admitted to a psychiatric hospital in an era when they were a relatively new phenomena in the mental health field. Since then, hospitals have continued to treat increasing numbers of adolescents, and some have begun to report their results. In addition, newer modalities of care and treatment have been introduced within the context of community mental health services, including shorter hospital stays and the use of residential facilities in the community, all aimed at reversing the regressive effects of institutionalization. At the same time, provision for lengthy hospitalization remains available on a selective basis for those adolescents requiring it.

Recently, many more young patients have been hospitalized for drug abuse and other problems, previously rare. Changing times bring changing problems and new challenges. Our increased knowledge of areas of strength, as well as of need, will, hopefully, place therapeutic resources in better perspective.

REFERENCES

1.   Hartmann, E., Glasser, B., Green-blatt, M., Solomon, M.H., and Levinson, D.J. Adolescents in a Mental Hospital. New York: Grune and Stratton, Inc., 1968.

Masterson, J. Prognosis in Adolescent Disorders. Amer. J. Psychiat. 114:1097-1103,1958.

Warren, W. A Study of Adolescent Psychiatric Inpatients and the Outcome Six or More Years Later: II. The Follow-up Study. J. of Child Psychology and Psychiatry. 6:141-160, 1965.

2.   Masterson, J. Prognosis in Adolescent Disorders. Amer. J. Psychiat. 114:1097-1103, 1958.

3. Warren, W. A Study of Adolescent
    Psychiatric Inpatients and the Out-
    come Six or More Years Later: II.
    The Follow-up Study. J. of Child
    Psychology and Psychiatry. 6:141-
    160, 1965.

4. Hartmann, E., Glasser, B., Green-
    blatt, M., Solomon, M.H., and Levin-
    son, D.J. Adolescents in a Mental
    Hospital. New York: Grune and
    Stratton, Inc., 1968.

5. Garber, B. Follow-up Study of Hospi-
    talized Adolescents. New York, Lon-
    don: Bruner/Mazel, 1972.

6. Ibid, p. 156

7. Hollingshead, A.B. and Redlich, F.C.
    Social Class and Mental Illness.
    New York: York & Wiley, 1958.

8. Hartmann, E., Glasser, B., Green-
    blatt, M., Solomon, M.H., and Levin-
    son, D.J. Adolescents in a Mental
    Hospital. New York: Grune and
    Stratton, Inc., 1968. p. 26.

9. Hartmann, E., Glasser, B. and Herrera,
    M.A. Adolescent Inpatients: Five
    Years Later. Seminars in Psychiatry.
    1:66-78, 1969. p. 68.

10. Hartmann, E., Glasser, B., Green-
    blatt, M., Solomon, M.H., and Levin-
    son, D.J. Adolescents in a Mental
    Hospital. New York: Grune and
    Stratton, Inc., 1968. p. 25.

11.   Hartmann, E., Glasser, B. and Herrera,
      M.A.   Adolescent Inpatients: Five
      Years Later.   Seminars in Psychiatry.
      1:66-78, 1969.   p. 75.

12.   Myers, J.K., and Bean, L.L.   A Decade
      Later: A Follow-up of Social Class
      and Mental Illness. New York, Lon-
      don, Sydney: John Wiley & Sons, Inc.,
      1968.

13.   Hollingshead, A.B. and Redlich, F.C.
      Social Class and Mental Illness.
      New York: York and Wiley, 1958.
      p. 342.

14.   Ibid, p. 342

15.   Ibid, p. 353

CHAPTER 9

EPILOGUE

Adolescents A Decade Later

At the time we had completed this
investigation, we had entered the decade
of the seventies. By now the mental
health professional had acquired considerable experience with the residential
treatment of adolescents, but the nature
of the problems and our own approaches to
treating them were evolving to such an extent that we could not conclude our work
without examining a 1970 adolescent population. We were interested to learn how
an adolescent entering a residential
treatment center almost a decade later
compared by way of his characteristics,
hospital experience, and outcome.

Meanwhile, McLean Hospital had been
consciously and continuously adjusting
to the many forces of change, both within
the hospital and in the community and
mental health field. Innovations in
psychiatric treatment came largely in new
arrangements (e.g., adolescent halls)
and diversity for the delivery of psychiatric care rather than in the development of completely new treatment methods.
Shorter term hospitalization had become a
trend, as well as the use of day care to

replace or supplement in-patient hospital-ization. In addition, the hospital had established its own halfway house and broken ground for the construction of an inpatient unit for children.

Within the hospital, there was a growing emphasis in all clinical depart-ments on the development of a wider range of skills by staff members, as well as an increased involvement of the patient in responsibility for his own treatment pro-gram. Considerable impetus was provided for the development of family, group and milieu therapies and rehabilitation. In-dividual therapy remained, notwith-standing, the major treatment modality.

The adolescents represented a signi-ficant component in the increasing admis-sion rate at the hospital. By 1970 patients under 20 years of age comprised 35 percent of the total admissions. De-spite the growing trend toward shorter hospitalization, adolescents were still in residence for extended stays.

The 1970 Investigation

The 1970 sample consisted of 65 patients, ranging in age from 13 through 19, and hospitalized for three months or more during the period from January 1, 1970 through November 30, 1970. Our ob-jectives included identifying this pop-ulation and their hospital experience, and carrying out a preliminary follow-up of them in January, 1973. A later follow-up of this group is projected at approxi-mately the five-year level to provide more reliable comparison with the earlier study.

Data collection was accomplished by
extraction of relevant information from
the medical records and intensive personal or telephone interviews, focusing on
the hospital experience and the post-
hospital adjustment. As in the earlier
study, both former patients and parents
were included as informants. In addition,
level of adjustment ratings of *mental
status* were obtained for the adolescents,
with consensus achieved by three independent raters, one of whom included the
interviewer who had conducted the follow-
up interview.

The first set of analyses involved
obtaining frequency distributions of the
major variables. Content analysis was
used to examine responses to open-ended
questions. A comparison was made of patient and relative responses. When purely
objective data were sought, information
was taken from the relatives' responses
(as in the "sixties" study) with the exception of some personal sections relating to the use of drugs and alcohol,
about which we felt the adolescents were
more knowledgable. Results of the 1970
study were examined to see if and how the
adolescent picture had altered over a
decade marked by rapid change in many
spheres.

Sample Characteristics. The 1970
sample was almost equally divided as to
sex, with slightly more females. The age
distribution was fairly even except for
very few 13 and 14 year olds. Approximately 11 percent of the patients were
adopted children, more than twice the
4.8 percent figure given in the census

report for the general population. The 11
percent adoption figure compares rather
closely with the 13 percent in the 1960
sample, making this particular characteristic one of the few in which the two
samples were similar.

The 1970 sample tended to come from
larger families. As many as 50 adolescents had two or more siblings, and there
was only one "only" child represented.
Birth order was evenly distributed, com-
prising more than twice as many "middle"
positions as in the earlier sample.

Religious affiliation was divided between Protestant, Catholic, and Jewish,
with nine adolescents stating they had
"no" religious preference. This represented a considerable drop in Protestant
patients and more than a doubling of Catholic patients, in contrast to the earlier
sample. The proportion of Jewish patients
remained high.

The area of education also reflected
the broadening population base from which
the McLean patients were now coming. The
majority of adolescents in the 1970 sample
had attended public secondary schools, a
sharp contrast to the predominantly private school education experienced by the
"sixties" sample patients.

Parents of the 1970 adolescents may
be characterized as well-educated, with a
clear majority having educational training
beyond the secondary level. Although similar in this respect to the "sixties" parents, they were reported to be more
"stable" in their marriages in contrast to

the earlier group for whom "some conflict"
in the marriage was noted with greater
frequency. In both samples, patient-
mother contact was described as "regular"
for almost all of the families; however,
patient-father contact was seen as "infrequent or alternating" for 18 percent
of the 1970 sample compared to 27 percent
of the "sixties" sample.

Hospitalization Data. For most of
the 1970 sample, this was the first admission to McLean Hospital. One half had
experienced previous hospitalization elsewhere, twice as many as in the earlier
sample. (This figure was affected to
some extent by the number of patients
placed elsewhere while on the McLean wait-
ing list). Also, 34 percent of the adolescents in 1970 had experienced a first
psychiatric contact before the age of 12,
somewhat higher than the 25 percent characterizing the "sixties" sample. These
statistics may be related to the pathology
in the later group, or reflect rather the
greater availability, use, and acceptance
of resources on its part.

More than twice as many patients were
admitted on court order, almost 21 percent
compared to 9 percent in the earlier decade - a figure somewhat reflecting the
drug phenomenon. Drug usage at the time
of admission was reported for at least 60
percent of the 1970 sample, a sharp increase over the 14 percent attributed to
the "sixties" adolescents. Although both
reported percentages are likely to be low,
there is unquestionably a sharp distinc-
tion between the two samples with respect
to this variable. It may well be one of

the major differences distinguishing them at admission.

Little emphasis has been placed in this work on diagnostic classifications because of variations among clinicians and in hospital philosophy influencing judgments. However, it may be useful to report a difference noted between the two populations. Although both were characterized as having two major classifications, schizophrenia and personality disorders (including adolescent adjustment reactions), the "sixties" sample had a greater number of personality disorders, by contrast with the 1970 sample which had more schizophrenics. This raised the possibility of an actual important difference in the two samples, but this question cannot be resolved because of other factors influencing the determination of diagnoses.

Although by 1970, many adolescents were receiving short-term hospitalization, this sample excluded all those hospitalized less than three months. Approximately half of both groups studied were hospitalized more than 300 days. Excluding the 17 in the 1970 sample who had not been fully discharged, the two samples were essentially identical with respect to condition at discharge: almost half of both samples were rated much or moderately improved.

With regard to destination at discharge, more patients in the 1970 sample went home (52 percent compared to 40 percent). Twenty percent of the earlier group were discharged to another psychiatric hospital, compared to 13 per-

cent of the 1970 group to date. Other
common destinations included halfway
houses, foster homes, residential schools,
and apartment settings.

        In summary, differences rather than
similarities characterized the two adolescents samples. The differences related in
varying respects to the following personal
and family variables: religious distribution, size of family, birth order, type
of education and marital adjustment of
parents. There were indications of clinical variations as well - previous psychiatric experience, diagnoses, and particularly the use of drugs prior to admission. Each group was exposed to long-
term private residential treatment at
McLean Hospital, having psychotherapy in
common as the major modality; however,
the programs differed in their level of
sophistication with respect to the management of adolescent problems and the
variety of therapeutic resources available.

        The Follow-up Experience. Inter-
viewing was carried out by 11 second-year
graduate students at the Simmons College
School of Social Work by means of a
structured interview schedule. The questionnaire was divided into several different sections relating to adjustment
with respect to personal, occupational,
social and family spheres of life, as
well as clinical and treatment status
and reactions to the hospitalization experience. A final section related to the
perceptions adolescents had of themselves
and of how their relatives saw them.

From a total sample population of 65,
follow-up information (minimally one
interview) was obtained for 56 patients
(86 percent of the sample). Three families refused to participate, and one
could not be reached. We did not approach
five former patients and their families
for follow-up because they had been involved in another recent hospital study,
and we felt that requesting research participation a second time was not justi-
fied. We were satisfied that these five
former patients were not unrepresentative
of the others for whom we had follow-up
data, either by way of the demographic and
hospital data characterizing them, or the
post-hospital adjustment data obtained
through a professional substitute, but not
included in the data analysis.

Parents participated in the follow-
up of all the 56 patients for whom we have
data: 40 mothers, and 27 fathers; 11 of
these were conjoint interviews. In addition, interviews were obtained from 47
adolescents. Parents refused us permission to contact 8 former patients; two
adolescents refused to participate, and
three were inaccessible.

Reactions to the follow-up interview
on the part of the 1970 families re-
affirmed our earlier experience with respect to the generally positive attitude
toward participation and a special respon-
siveness to the hospital's interest in
learning how they had been doing. Many
expressed satisfaction at the opportunity
afforded either to praise or criticize the
hospital. One particular difference between the two studies pleased us. Al-

though in the "sixties" study there were
only 24 former patients interviewed (most
often because of refusal on the part of
family to give permission, or inaccessibility), in the 1970 study twice as many
were seen, and all of them had a parent
participating as well. The 47 parent-
adolescent combination interviews provided us a good opportunity to compare
adolescent and parent views of current
progress and the treatment experience.

Comparison of Outcome of the Two Samples

A comparison of outcome of the two
groups must be viewed here as suggestive
rather than definitive because of the time
interval when follow-up took place; for
the "sixties" sample it was an average of
4 years after discharge, or 5.5 after admission, compared to 1.5 average years
after discharge, or 2.5 after admission,
for the 1970 sample. The average age at
follow-up for the earlier sample was 23.3
years, contrasted with 19.4 for the 1970
sample. Our earlier investigation had
postulated that the adaptation of the former to the stresses of life seemed to improve somewhat as he matured. We were also impressed at the five-year follow-up
by the tendency for either improvement or
decline to have been sustained for a period of time. An examination of the 1970
outcome at an earlier point in time appeared promising, in terms of the emerging trends which would be delineated.

Outcome data were compared in both
samples with respect to several selected
variables in an effort to elicit similarities or differences. There was an immed-

iately important difference in the *mental status* ratings of the two samples. In the earlier investigation, 37 individuals were rated as GOOD; 8, FAIR; and 11, POOR. The 1970 sample had 20 with GOOD ratings; 30, FAIR: and 3, POOR. Even though both groups had improved at the time of follow-up, GOOD *mental status* ratings dominated the long-term follow-up sample by contrast with FAIR *mental status* ratings for the 1970 sample. Also of interest was the difference in POOR ratings; the "sixties" sample had more than three times the number of the 1970 group. These figures would confirm the observation noted of a trend toward either end of the *mental status* ratings continuum.

Marital Status. As would have been anticipated, almost all of the 1970 population were unmarried at the time of follow-up. Two had married, but both were already in the process of seeking divorces. The higher percentage of married subjects in the earlier study reflects the difference in the follow-up interval, as well as the more prevalent occurrence today of couples living together without legal sanction.

Residence. The type of residence of former patients was used as a variable for comparison. The 1970 sample at follow-up had a fairly even distribution of those living independently (i.e., alone, with friends, with spouse), with parents, or in some treatment facility. Residence at follow-up compared with destination at discharge had shown a shift away from living with parents to more independent arrangements, with a somewhat lower num-

ber in residential settings. This progression away from parents and residential
treatment settings had also characterized
the "sixties" subjects, who were living
independently at follow-up, with the exception of a small minority. Of particular interest is the mobility which
characterized both groups and the trend in
both samples away from parental and treatment settings to independent living
arrangements.

School and Work. Eighty-nine percent
of the adolescents hospitalized in 1970
were at school or working at follow-up,
compared to 73 percent of the adolescents
in the earlier investigation. This would
appear to be rather striking evidence of
occupational activity on the part of the
1970 sample, particularly in view of the
fact that as many as nine young people
were hospitalized at the time of the investigation.

A similar difference in the two
groups was observed with respect to
schooling since discharge; approximately
75 percent of the 1970 population had some
schooling after hospital discharge, compared to 57 percent of the earlier study.
At the time of follow-up, thirty-two of
the 1970 adolescents were attending school,
the majority reported doing well and "enjoying it". As many as 34 in this sample
had work experience following hospital discharge, with 18 working at the time of
follow-up. The kinds of jobs held varied
widely, although most were in the un-
skilled or semi-unskilled variety. Again,
a majority of those employed were seen as
making an adequate adjustment in this area;

many expressed hopes for a variety of vocational careers, ranging from dreams of
adventure and success to service-oriented
goals.

The area of school-work conveys a
fairly promising level of adaptation at
follow-up for the 1970 population. Although both samples were dissimilar in
many ways, no special qualities of this
group would have led us to predict this.
In the earlier investigation, the adolescents experienced a fair amount of occupational difficulties over the post-
hospital years with a trend toward increasing mastery with maturation, for
those who were improving. For a smaller
number, failure in this area became more
evident; apparently, the inroads of the
illness tend to impose a particular strain
on the vocational capacities of the individual, a fact which is complicated by
the attitudes of prospective employers
toward the mentally ill.

It is possible to consider that we
are experiencing the impact of increasingly successful school programming and
vocational counseling in the residential
treatment setting. If the adjustment
achieved in this area is maintained or increased at the five year level of follow-
up, we would have some reason to believe
that rehabilitative intervention had taken
place.

Self-Management. Adolescents in the
1970 sample were for the most part still
financially dependent on their parents at
follow-up, as would be expected from so
young a group. Approximately one-fourth,

however, were already supporting themselves, partially or mainly. In the
earlier investigation, almost one-half
were responsible for their self-support,
with the rest still requiring subsidi-
zation, or complete support, from parents.

Another area in which the 1970 adolescent was reported to be making strides
was that of assuming household responsibilities; he was viewed at follow-up as
having more household tasks than at hospital admission, and as being more apt to
fulfill them.

In both studies, the area of self-
management, particularly as it relates to
financial independence, was not considered
a major criterion of the level of post-
hospital adjustment at follow-up because
of the relatively young age of the sample
population. There has been a general recognition in the last decade not only of
the lowered age of puberty but also of the
prolongation of adolescence, largely as a
result of higher education as an expectation, and the financial dependence it
usually entails. Some writers have suggested that it may extend to the age of
twenty-three. An additional factor with
this particular group of young people is
the disruption inherent in a serious illness occurring during this period. An
examination of this population ten years
after hospitalization would provide important information about the level of
maturity with respect to self-management
achieved by the formerly hospitalized
adolescent as an older adult.

Relationship with Parents. Separation from parents has been acknowledged as
a basic life task of the adolescent years.
While this can be a turbulent period for
many adolescents and their families, a genuine concern about their relationship
with parents is often at the same time
characteristic of the adolescent period.
Our adolescents were no exceptions to
these trends; they were, if anything, just
more so.

An important but expected difference
between the samples emerged here. As has
been documented earlier, improvement in
relationships with parents in the earlier
population was a meaningful ingredient of
the adjustment experience at follow-up.
This appeared to be related to increased
understanding, geographical separation,
and maturation. As expected, at follow-
up, the younger 1970 population was still
involved in a struggle to develop more
satisfying ties with parents, particularly
mother. Some improvement was noted, however, particularly in relationship with
father. This is consistent with an earlier observation in our study that improvement in relationship with father
occurred at a more accelerated rate between hospital admission and discharge
than did improvement in relationship with
mother. Adjustment to mother was reported
to have achieved statistical significance
with respect to the level of functioning
only at the five-year follow-up. This
would lead us to anticipate that further
gains will be achieved in this area, with
subsequent improvement in general functioning anticipated as well.

Of interest to us was the recurrent
refrain from those interviewed in the
recent sample who attributed gains made in
their relationships with each other to the
increased understanding and self-awareness
resulting from therapeutic intervention.

Social Relationships. With respect
to the social life of the former patients,
considerably fewer in the 1970 sample (in
contrast to the earlier population) may
be characterized as being isolated, a
rather interesting finding for a group
with predominantly schizophrenic diagnoses.
The relationship with peers included the
same and opposite sex, with dating reported for 60 percent. The large majority
were described as having people in their
lives who could be called "friends".
Reading, music, and movies were recreational interests described with the most
frequency, with movies being the major
activity with friends.

Whether the lesser social activity of
the "sixties" sample is related to the
post-hospital interval, and increasing
pathology of some former patients, or to
other factors is not clear. For one
thing, the current generation of adolescents may exhibit more group-mindedness
and acceptance of each other than in the
earlier decade. There is evidence to
suggest that the young patient entering
a residential treatment setting today
feels less "stigmatized" than his counter-
part in the early sixties. Much of the
content in the follow-up interviews
carried out in the later study provided
such references.

It is also possible that the current emphasis in hospital programming on milieu modalities as a serious addition to the traditional intensive psychotherapy which provided the main therapeutic avenue in the early sixties, has had positive reper- cussions in the area of the patient's social life.

Clinical Status. At follow-up, 9 of the 1970 adolescent population were in psychiatric hospitals, and eight more were on-visit status at McLean, not yet dis- charged, although in the community. More than one-half of the discharged patients were receiving some form of treatment, most often psychotherapy. The next most common type of treatment was psychotropic medication, followed by group therapy and by administrative interviews. Many young people were receiving combinations of the modalities enumerated. Hospital read- missions had been experienced by twenty percent of the adolescents who had been discharged or were on-visit status.

These adolescents, as a group, were seen as doing better than at the time of admission, despite the fact that they were still struggling with basic issues around which they had been hospitalized. Recogni- tion was given to new successes in school, maintaining relationships with friends, and developing more confidence in the ability to make independent decisions, but the adolescents were still burdened with problems in areas such as family and social life, achieving independence, and mastery over emotional ups and downs. Moderate to extreme dissatisfaction with

current functioning was voiced by those
who revealed real skepticism as to the
permanency of the emotional changes
achieved.

Roughly the same number of individuals in both samples continued treatment
immediately after discharge from the hospital. The earlier group had shown, however,
a greater number returning to treatment
during the first six-month post-hospital
period than the 1970 sample. The smaller
percentage of hospital readmissions noted
for the recent population is, to some extent, a function of the shorter post-
hospital interval; however, it is of interest that in both samples, rehospital-
ized patients came from all *mental status*
groupings.

In summary, a comparison of outcome of
the two samples was limited by the difference in the average age of the adolescents and in the distance from the hospital experience. Also, both samples were
shown to be more unlike than alike at admission, and to have had different residential treatment experiences. However,
several rather interesting and similar
patterns emerged for both samples. For
one thing, improvement characterized the
outcome of both groups, as evidenced both
by subjective feelings of progress made
and level of adjustment achieved in certain areas. Differences between the
samples related more often to degree than
to actual dissimilarities. Both reported
improved ties with parents, yet there was
strong evidence that former patients in
the 1970 sample were experiencing considerably more frustration in this area,

particularly with respect to mother. The
gradual shift away from living with parents
and from residential settings was much
greater in the long-term sample, as would
be anticipated, but the direction was the
same for both samples. All former patients were assuming increasing financial
and household responsibilities, as be-
fitting their age and needs. The level of
adjustment with respect to social and
occupational roles appeared promising for
the 1970 sample, and the potential impact
of current educational and rehabilitative
resources is considered one possible explanation.

It was also shown that many former
patients continued to use psychiatric
services in the post-hospital period with
occasional rehospitalization when necessary. Use of resources varied from intermittent to continuous, with a small number
for whom hospitalization at the time of
follow-up was indicative of more serious
illness.

Drug Usage: 1970 Sample

The 1970 questionnaire contained two
sections not included in the earlier
study: questions relating to drug usage
and to the adolescent's self-image and
parents' perceptions of him. The follow-
up interviews revealed that as many as 72
percent of the adolescent sample were
using drugs at admission, (a large but
not unexpected increase over the 14 percent noted in the "sixties" sample). Evidence of drug usage was included for any
admitted use of a particular drug,
irrespective of the extent to which it was

used. This high percentage was derived
primarily from the heavy use of marijuana,
reportedly used to the same degree following hospitalization. A decrease in the
use of LSD, amphetamines, and heroin was
noted, while marijuana, as mentioned,
barbiturates and other drugs continued to
be used to much the same degree. Heavy
usage of drugs was defined as either daily
use of a particular drug or the frequent
and continued use of several drugs over a
period of time. Twenty-two former patients were seen as heavy drug users before their hospitalization, while nine
were reported to be heavy users after
discharge.

Self-Image and Parental Perceptions:
1970 Sample

        The adolescent was asked to describe
himself at admission and at the time of
follow-up, and how he thought his parents
viewed him at these two points in time.
Parents were also requested to give their
perceptions of the adolescent, again for
both time intervals. We were hopeful that
their responses would be useful indicators
of perceptual and behavioral change, as
well as clues to the correspondence of
feelings between parent and child.

        Ninety percent of the adolescents,
and a corresponding 90 percent of the
parents, had a negative or critical view
of the patient at admission, and adolescents predicted accurately that 90 percent of their parents had such a perception. Again, there was a degree of
similarity in how the young person saw
himself at the time of follow-up and how

his parent viewed him; 65 percent of the
adolescents saw themselves in positive
terms, compared to 59 percent of the parents. However, adolescents had predicted
that 72 percent of the parents would view
them positively. Therefore, we found that
both former patient and the parent were
completely in agreement in their negative
perceptions of the adolescent at the time
of hospitalization, but the adolescent now
viewed himself somewhat more positively
than his parent viewed him, and over-
estimated his parent's current view of
him.

Of more significance was the extent
to which the perceptions had changed -
from 90 percent of the adolescents at
hospital admission characterized as "suicidal" - "sick" - "hostile" - "burned-up"-
"crazy on drugs", etc., to more than 60
percent who were later viewed as "coping"-
"mature" - "growing" - "confident" - "all-
right", etc. One-third of the adolescents
still saw themselves, however, as "lonely"-
"desperate" - "manipulative" - "a loser",
etc.; while two-fifths of the parents
used such terms as "unrealistic" - "de-
manding" - "unpredictable" - "lost", etc.,
to describe their offspring. But, for
the majority, the direction had been
positive.

Comparison cf Adolescent and Parent
Responses

The 47 combination interviews of
adolescent and parent permitted a comparison of the way in which the two evaluated
current functioning. Ratings of adolescents and parents reflect similar direc-

tion, but with some differences in degree. The adolescent tended to regard himself as somewhat better than his parent saw him in his social relationships, work situations, and emerging financial independence; however, with regard to school, his household responsibilities, and relationship to mother, he saw less progress than the parent. He was clearly more knowledgeable about his use of drugs. In practically all cases where parent and child responses did not correlate, it was the parent who indicated the drug had not been used, while the child reported it had been. Parents, thus, appeared to be either uninformed or unrealistic about the extent to which their offspring were using drugs.

Agreement was relatively close between the adolescent and his parent about his clinical status, although the adolescent's estimate of progress and of his parent's perception of how well he was doing, tended to be slightly higher than the parent's evaluation.

It is possible that these variations relate to the different value systems of the two generations, and their respective expectations.

Reactions to the Hospitalization:
1970 Sample

The hospital stay was viewed positively or with mixed feeling, for the most part. (Negative feelings were reported by 19 percent of the adolescents, 7 percent of the parents). A closer examination of the reactions to many aspects of the experience provided a better understanding of satisfaction and dissatisfaction.

Satisfaction was mainly attributed to increased insight on the part of the adolescent and better understanding of his problem. In addition, the majority of parents felt that the hospitalization had served to affect their own self-awareness, with resultant improvement in their individual functioning and in family interaction.

Criticism was directed at management issues (degree of permissiveness, length of stay, etc.), psychotherapy, communication, medication and staffing. Some attention was given to the need for change in such specific areas as locked halls, food, and cost of hospitalization. Former patients tended to be more critical than their parents, in all areas, but, on the whole, reactions were similar.

Therapy, and the therapist, emerged as important factors in the total experience. This was evidenced not only by the rating of "helpful" often given to the professional, but also by the acknowledgement of increased insight and understanding attributed to the therapeutic relationship. Among those adolescents who did not find therapy helpful were those who felt they had not used therapy properly.

However, frustrations, particularly on the part of the former patient, were experienced in relation to what was described as the inaccessibility of the psychiatrist-administrator. By contrast, satisfaction with nurses, and especially

the psychiatric aides, seemed to reflect
that their roles offer greater opportunity
for contact and communication. The social
worker was viewed as having helped to
facilitate communication between the
adolescent and his family, but as being
less helpful to the patient himself. The
Arlington School experience was invariably
considered to be highly meaningful and
valuable, very often because of the quality of relationship between the educational staff and former patient.

Expectations from the hospital experience included cure, relief of symptoms,
relief of home tensions, and prevention of
further progression of symptoms. Almost
one-half felt that the hospital had met
some of their expectations. Of more moment, was the reporting of a development
of understanding in the course of hospitalization that the original expectation
(i.e., for a cure) was unrealistic, and a
growing acceptance of lesser but attain-
able goals.

Community reactions to "the hospitalization" did not appear to be a
serious issue for this population, although approximately one-third experienced stigma in social or vocational
situations, or with other family members.
Although the fact of hospitalization was
usually shared with other family members,
the former patient was more sensitive than
his parent about revealing it; approximately 28 percent compared to 9 percent
felt unable to do so.

In comparing the reactions of the
two populations studied, we were impressed

with a strong difference. Despite the
candid quality of all informants, and the
ease with which they were able to discuss
criticisms and disappointments, there
emerged in the 1970 population by contrast
with the earlier one, a clear affirmation
of the helpfulness of the overall experience and its therapeutic input. The
data are presumptive that our accumulative
experience with hospitalized adolescents
over the decade has resulted in more effective methods of patient care. It is
also possible that the former patients'
and families' retrospective view of hospitalization is affected by the perspective
of distance from time of discharge; distance from the experience may blur the
sharpness of impact.

Retrospect and Outlook

    Hospitalization for the seriously
disturbed adolescent in the early sixties,
though often a last resort, was the only
hope or refuge for him and his anguished
family. In the intervening years, the
popularization of more varied life styles
among the young has created a climate of
greater tolerance for deviant behavior.
New outlets were found in communal living
arrangements, religious cults, and mysti-
cal movements. Not only were new avenues
provided for the sheltering of those with
non-conformist or unconventional behavior,
but the general community also seemed more
receptive to "difference".

    At the same time, in keeping with the
needs of the population seeking psychiatric hospitalization, many private hospitals were diversifying their programs with

many possible arrangements for care: short
or long-term residential treatment, day
and night care, after-care, school programs, and half-way houses. Specialized
facilities were often added for treatment
of drug abuse and alcoholism. An increasing variety of specific treatment
modalities geared to the particular needs
of the patient became available, with
treatment no longer limited to him but
extended to the family unit. Early return to the community became emphasized
nation-wide, and community services pro-
liferated.

It is reasonable to anticipate that
presenting problems and treatment needs
will continue to evolve in the context
of societal change, and that we will continue to need adequate residential care
for the seriously ill. It is also increasingly evident that as a way of moni-
toring changes and program effectiveness,
evaluative research offers hope that our
knowledge and resources will keep pace
with the developing needs. Many hospitals
are moving in the direction of including
evaluation in their programming and in
assuming responsibility for the imple-
mentation of findings. For example, on-
going follow-up programs for all discharged
patients are being encouraged; in some
settings, an innovative approach to more
relevant data collection is made possible
by the new problem-oriented record system
being adopted.

The documentation of our experiences
in a decade of work with adolescents is
but a beginning step. Further work is
indicated and projected for the future:

the five-year follow-up of the 1970 investigation, a ten-year investigation to
assess this population as older adults,
and control studies of comparable groups
who have not undergone hospitalization.

Thus far, our findings give us reason
to be hopeful about the outlook for the
hospitalized adolescent. Continued efforts at integrating evaluative data
with new systems and modalities of care
will help to assure that his transition
from hospital to community will hold more
enduring promise for a better life.

CODE   OUTLINE

1. Preadmission Data
   A. The Patient
      1. Sex
      2. Birthdate
      3. Marital status
      4. Age at time of marriage
      5. Religion
      6. Birthplace
   B. Education
      1. Grade Level completed
      2. Grade level of first school difficulty
      3. Did Patient leave school? Why?
      4. Type of schooling (primary and secondary)
      5. Number of schools (primary and secondary
      6. Academic performance (primary and secondary)
      7. Variability of performance (primary and secondary)
      8. Post-secondary education (type, level, performance)

Note: Outline form does not give the number of possible answers for each item. Range from 2 to 20.

C. Social Relations
    1. Friendships (sex, age, fre-
        quency)
    2. Dating patterns
D. Extra-curricular activities -
    degree of involvement in:
    1. Athletics
    2. Arts
    3. Hobbies
    4. Organizations
E. Preadmission behavior problems
    (Ratings on when and if 63 pro-
    blems appeared)
F. Psychiatric History
    (Number, place, and time, of fre-
    quency and mode of previous treat-
    ments)
G. Medical History
    (Birth defects, accidents, ill-
    nesses. Age of onset, length
    of treatment, etc.)
H. Family History
    1. Who are "focal parents"
    2. Natural parents - for each
        parent:
        a. Life status (if dead,
            age of patient when
            death occurred)
        b. Religion
        c. Education
        d. Marital status (at pa-
            tient's birth, at
            time of death, at
            time of critical ad-
            mission)
        e. Occupation
        f. Illnesses and injuries
    3. Siblings
        a. Number of siblings
        b. Number of natural sib-
            lings older and
            younger of each sex

c. Number of adopted
    siblings and half-
    siblings, older and
    younger of each sex
d. Age differences of
    next older and
    younger siblings
e. Multiple births
f. Miscarriages, still-
    births, abortions of
    mother
g. Injuries and deaths
    of siblings
h. Marriage history of
    siblings
4. Parent surrogates
    All of the data obtained
    for natural parents is re-
    corded here for adoptive
    or step-parents, plus:
    age at adoption
5. Surrogate family siblings
    All of the data obtained
    previously for siblings
    is recorded here if pa-
    tient had both natural
    family and surrogate
    family
I. Residential History
    1. Type and duration of pre-
        vious living arrangements
    2. "Significant others" living
        with patient
    3. Number of living arrange-
        ments in last three years
    4. Age at which patient first
        left home
    5. Separations of patient from
        mother and father
        a. Frequency
        b. Reasons
        c. Age

6. Early childhood living
    arrangements (type, num-
    ber of moves, significant
    others, patient-mother
    contact, mother substi-
    tutes)

J. Parents Presentation of Problems
    1. Description of which of 16
        problems the patient's
        focal mother presented
        to the social worker
    2. Description of which of 16
        problems the patient's
        focal father presented
        to the social worker
    3. Where parents see cause of
        problem (each parent)
        a. Patient himself, emo-
            tionally and/or
            physically
        b. Patient's family
        c. Environment
    4. Relationship of parents to
        patient's problems
        a. Their attempts to
            deal with the pro-
            blems
        b. Their social acknow-
            ledgement of the
            problems
        c. Their hopes of accom-
            plishment through
            hospitalization
        d. Their concepts of
            effect of problems
            on their marital
            relations

K. Social worker's impressions of
    parents' relation to patient.
    Ratings of mother's and father's
    reactions to patient along nine
    (9) dimensions.

L.   Family history of psychiatric
     contact. Who in family has had
     treatment and for what problems?
M.   Early childhood experiences
     1.   Mother's pregnancy -
          physical or psychologi-
          cal problems
     2.   Problems in delivering baby
     3.   Status of baby at birth
     4.   Child's development (rate
          of physical development,
          verbal development, and
          toilet training)

II. Hospitalization Data
    A.   Referral Behavior - presence or
         absence of 62 behavior problems
    B.   Critical statistics
         1.   Date of admission
         2.   Age at admission
         3.   Length of time hospital-
              ized and time in resi-
              dence
         4.   Date and age at discharge
         5.   Number of previous McLean
              admissions
         6.   Total length of time pre-
              viously at McLean
         7.   Source of referral and
              first contact
         8.   Age of mother and surro-
              gate mother at admission
         9.   Age of father and surro-
              gate father at admission
         10. Who accompanied patient on
              admission
         11. Source of payment
         12. Patient's reaction to ad-
              mission (cooperative,
              anxious, etc.

13. Legal status of patient at admission
14. Events leading to admission (court order, school, acute episode, etc.)
15. Precipitating event

C. Visits During Hospitalization
1. Patient's visits - number, length
2. Visits by mother and/or mother surrogate and/or father and/or father surrogate. Number and rate
3. Number of escapes and for how many days

D. Extra-curricular Activities During Admission
Rate of involvement in sports, the arts, hobbies and organizations

E. Social Relations During Hospitalization
1. Rate of involvement with friends of same sex
2. Rate of involvement with friends of opposite sex
3. Age range of friends of each sex
4. Residence of friends (in or out of hospital)
5. Patient's participation in hospital activities (job, occupational therapy, recreational therapy, clubs, trips, etc.)
6. Dating pattern during hospitalization
7. Age of dating partners during hospitalization

F. Education During Hospitalization
        1. Type of program, if any
        2. Length of time between ad-
            mission and start of
            school
        3. Number of semesters en-
            rolled
        4. Absences
        5. Academic performance and
            variability of per-
            formance
        6. Number of school grades
            completed
        7. Reason for termination
G. Social Work
        1. Number of social workers
        2. How soon after admission
            social work began
        3. For each social worker:
            length of contact, fre-
            quency of contact with
            patient, with parents
            and combined, frequency
            of contact with other
            relatives
        4. Nature of problems ex-
            plored with social
            worker (which problems
            explored and with whom)
        5. Patient's attitude toward
            social work
        6. Parents' attitude toward
            social work
        7. Patient's and parents'
            goals for social work
        8. Reasons for termination of
            social work (each of
            these items was deter-
            mined for each social
            worker involved)

H. Therapy
    1.   Number of therapists
    2.   How soon after admission was first therapist seen?
    3.   For each therapist: length of contact, frequency of contact, reasons for change in therapist, areas explored in therapy, etc.

I. Hospital Residences
    1.   Number of halls
    2.   Which halls
    3.   Length of time in each hall
    4.   Number of roommates in each hall
    5.   Reason for change from each hall
    6.   Effect of change from each hall

J. Termination of Hospitalization
    1.   Who terminated hospitalization? (hospital, patient, family, etc.)
    2.   Proposed destination
    3.   Actual destination
    4.   Treatment plan (setting, therapist, type of treatment)
    5.   Discharge diagnosis
    6.   Estimate of progress
        a. Therapist
        b. Hall staff
        c. Social worker
    7.   Prognosis for patient
        a. Therapist
        b. Hall staff
        c. Social worker

III. Follow-up Data
    A. Follow-up Interview
          1.   Number of interviews
          2.   Informant(s)
          3.   Time between critical admission and discharge to interview
          4.   Length and setting of interview
          5.   Time and frequency and quality of informant's contact with patient
    B. Psychiatric Contact Since Discharge
          1.   First contact - time, nature, length
          2.   Number of contacts and number of hospitalizations
          3.   Time spent cumulatively in hospitals since discharge
          4.   Total number of therapists and time spent cumulatively in therapy
          5.   Time at McLean Hospital since discharge
          6.   Parents' psychiatric contacts since discharge
    C. Changes in Status Since Discharge
          1.   Marital status
               a.   Mother, adoptive mother, stepmother
               b.   Father, adoptive father, stepfather
          2.   Deaths since discharge (and cause of)
               a.   Patient (and age of)
               b.   Focal mother (patient's age at time of)
               c.   Focal father (pa-

                              tient's age at
                              time of)
                        d.   Siblings
D.   Problems in Patient's Family
     Since Discharge
          1.   Non-hospitalized emotional
          2.   Hospitalized - emotional
          3.   Alcoholism
          4.   Drug problem
E.   Schooling
          1.   School completed by dis-
                charge
          2.   Type and number of schools
                since discharge
          3.   Graduation since discharge
          4.   Post-high education since
                discharge
          5.   Performance and variability
                of performance in school
                since discharge
          6.   Current condition at school
F.   Residential History
          1.   Number and average length
                of residences since
                discharge
          2.   Type and length of each
                residence
          3.   Reason for change from each
                residence
G.   Work History
          1.   Current employment and/or
                work history
          2.   Number and average length
                of jobs since discharge
          3.   Estimate of functioning
                at job
          4.   Current condition at job
H.   Family History
          1.   Current marital status
          2.   Number and length of pre-
                vious marriages

3. Pregnancy at time of
    marriage(s)
4. Number of children,
    adopted or natural, from
    each marriage. (dept.
    released, uncleased, etc.)
5. Number of children
    currently with patient
6. Present pregnancy
7. Present attachment to
    children
8. If currently married:
    a. Informant's view of
        spouse and quality
        of relationship
    b. Informant's view of
        effect of marriage
        and psychiatric
        status

I. Financial Arrangements
    1. Source
    2. Effective management
J. Patient's Independence and
    Autonomy
K. Social Reactions (current and
    while at McLean)
    1. Association with peers
    2. Dating pattern
    3. Extra-curricular activities
        (sports, church, art,
        drama, music, social
        groups, other)
L. Changes in Behavior of Mother
    and Father to Patient and Reasons
    for Changes
    1. Disciplinary management
    2. Supervisory management
    3. Acceptance
M. Informant's View of Patient's
    Current Condition
    1. As compared with time of
        admission

2. Relationship with mother (or surrogate)
3. Relationship with father (or surrogate)

N. Attitudes Toward Hospital
   1. Who was most helpful?
   2. Did the hospital take over parental authority
   3. Hospital action regarding parental visiting
   4. Inconsistency in hospital management
   5. Reaction to management changes
   6. Problems about restrictions (or lack of)
   7. Effect of associations (peer and/or older patients)
   8. Contact with therapist (effect of and satisfaction)
   9. Contact with social worker (effect of and satisfaction)
   10. Contact with nurses (effect of and satisfaction)
   11. General reaction to hospitalization
   12. Report of lack of communication with hospital and/or doctors

O. Informant's Presentation of Patient's Problems
   1. Number of Problems
   2. Which of 16 problems were presented, and whether problems were current and/or past

P. Informant's View of Changes
    Produced by Hospitalization
        1. Therapeutic changes
        2. Ameliorative changes
        3. Changes informant wished
            hospital had produced
Q. Interviewer's impression of in-
    formant's attitude toward pa-
    tient ratings on 26 variables
    (empathy, anxiety, hostility,
    etc.)
R. Interviewer's Rating of Inter-
    view
        1. Ratings of informant's
            behavior
            a. Anxiety
            b. Cooperation
            c. Optimism
        2. Main areas of discussion
            in interview
        3. Estimate of informant's
            motivation for partici-
            pation in the study

.

VARIABLES EXCLUDED - INSIGNIFICANT DATA
(Data Not Available for
at Least 30 Percent of the Sample)

	% No Data
Title	

PREADMISSION VARIABLES

Title	% No Data
Patient's Involvement in Religion	64.2
Area of Specialization in College	89.5
Patient's Involvement in Sports	31.3
Frequency of Contact With Major Professional at Second Psychiatric Contact	53.8
Natural Mother's Involvement in Religion	73.1
Natural Father's Involvement in Religion	76.1
Natural Mother's Occupation Before Assuming Household Duties	65.7
Who Cared for Patient in Absence of Mother	40.3
Mother's Physical Problems With Pregnancy of Patient	35.8
Mother's Problems Associated with Birth of Patient	32.8

HOSPITALIZATION VARIABLES

Title	% No Data
Months From Admission to Start of School	42.9

Title	% No Data
HOSPITALIZATION VARIABLES (continued)	
Frequency of Absence From School During Hospitalization	63.1
Variability of Academic Performance	44.9
#Grades Completed During Hospitalization	53.1
How Did Patient's School Program Terminate	81.6
Frequency of Social Worker Telephone Contact With Mother and Father	32.2
How Did Total Social Work Experience Terminate	33.3
How Long Did Total Social Work Experience Last	37.3
Effect of Change From First Hall	38.6
Total Number of Roommates on Second Hall	77.3
Effect of Change From Second Hall	55.9
Planned Mode of Treatment After Discharge	47.6
Therapist's Estimate of Patient's Progress	84.1
Social Worker's Estimate of Patient's Progress	84.1
Therapist's Prognosis	86.7
Staff's Prognosis	66.7
Social Worker's Prognosis	85.7
Illnesses During Hospitalization	59.7
Mother's Illnesses or Accidents	96.8
Father's Illnesses or Accidents	90.5
Siblings Illnesses or Accidents	90.5
Family - Non-Hospitalized Mental or Emotional Treatment	52.4
Family - Hospitalized Mental or Emotional Treatment	52.4

	% No Data
Title	

HOSPITALIZATION VARIABLES (continued)

Family - Non-Institutionalized Mental Deficiency	52.4
Family - Hospitalized Mental Deficiency	52.4
Family - Alcoholism	52.4
Family - Drug or Narcotic Abuse	52.4
Relationship to Mom - Discharge Rating	58.3
Relationship to Dad - Discharge Rating	62.3
Relationship to Peers - Discharge Rating	79.4
Relationship to Work-School - Discharge Rating	49.2

FOLLOW-UP VARIABLES

Undergraduate Study Program Since Discharge	39.4
Professional Degree Objectives	42.4
Variability of College Performance	60.6
# Months at 2nd Living Arrangement	36.7
# Times 'To go away from' Reason For Change	41.7
# Times 'To go to' Something Reason for Change	41.7
# Times 'To go to own place' Reason for Change	35.0

APPENDIX C

LEVEL OF ADJUSTMENT RATINGS*

1. Mental Status
          Good   Fair   Poor

    AREAS CONSIDERED:
    A.   Formal Mental Status (Appear-
         ance and behavior, reality
         orientation, mood, specific
         symptoms)
    B.   Responsibility for Behavior
         (delinquency, sexual impulses,
         agressive impulses)
    C.   Self (ambitions, interests,
         energy, initiative, self-eval-
         uation and responsibility for
         self, awareness of others,
         capacity for mature, mutual
         relationships)

    RATINGS:
    GOOD: No significant pathology in
           any area, i.e. all three areas
           are rated Good.
    FAIR: At least one rating of moder-
           ate pathology, but no more

---

*This rating scale was taken directly
from Hartmann, E., et. al., Adolescents in
a Mental Hospital, Grune and Stratton,
Inc., New York, 1968. pp. 143-146.

than one rating of severe
pathology in the three areas.

POOR: A rating of severe pathology -
Poor in two or three areas.

2. The Patient's relationship With His
Family of Orientation:

	a. Mother		b. Father
Good		Fair	Poor

GOOD: A stable relationship, demon-
strating mutual respect and at
least some affection.

FAIR: Relationship clearly impaired.
No attempt is made to assess
how much of this might be
attributable to the patient
rather than his family.

POOR: The relationship is totally
or preponderantly void of the
qualities rated Good.

3. Relationship With Peers

	Good	Fair	Poor

GOOD: At least one mutual, gratifying relationship with a peer
of either sex. Relationships
with other peers of both sexes
are not grossly restricted.

FAIR: Clear evidence of gross re-
striction in some aspect of
relationships with peers. Relationships to groups but not
to individuals.

POOR: No friends at all, or only
superficial acquaintance with
schoolmates or fellow workers,
or, for those now in hospital,
only superficial acquaintance
with other patients.

4. <u>Work-School</u>
         Good   Fair   Poor

   GOOD: Attends work or school with
          some measure of stability or
          success.
   FAIR: Significant problems in school
          or work. (Truancy, acting out,
          etc.)
   POOR: Unable or unwilling to attend
          school or work.

APPENDIX D
Data Summaries, 1970 Sample
(65 Patients)

Sex

Males	Females
30	35

Age

13-14	15	16	17	18	19
3	12	11	14	10	15

Siblings

0	1	2	3	4 or more
1	14	23	14	13

Birth Order

Youngest	Middle	Oldest
21	22	22

Religion

None	Catholic	Protestant	Jewish
9	16	20	20

Type of High School Education

Public	Private	Public & Private	Inapplicable or No Data
27	9	13	16

Marital Adjustment

	Stable	Some Conflict	Inapplicable or No Data
As described by Mother	30	28	7
As described by Father	33	28	4

Early Child Contact

	Regular	Fluctuating or Infrequent	Inapplicable or No Data
With Mother	59	5	1
With Father	49	11	4

APPENDIX D (continued)

Discharge Diagnosis

Schizophrenia	Personality Disorders	Other
28	19	1

Length of Hospitalization (in days)

100	101-200	201-300	301-400	401+
4	16	15	6	24 (17 not yet discharged)

Mental Status Ratings at Follow-up

Good	Fair	Poor	Inapplicable or No Data
20	30	3	12

Residence at Follow-up

Parent's or Friend's Home	Apartment Home	Dormitory	Halfway House	Treatment Facility	Inapplicable or No Data
16	14	7	7	11	10

Occupational Activity at Follow-up

Primarily at School	Primarily at Work	No Activity	Inapplicable or No Data
32	18	5	10

Relationship with Mother at Follow-up

	Good	Fair	Poor	Inapplicable or No Data
(Relative's report)	34	14	5	12
(Patient's report)	16	15	13	20

APPENDIX D (continued)

Relationship with Father at Follow-up	Good	Fair	Poor	Inapplicable or No Data
(Relative's report)	30	14	5	16
(Patient's report)	21	15	9	20

Social Relationships at Follow-up	Some or Many Friends	No Friends	Inapplicable or No Data
	47	6	12

Treatment at Follow-up*	None	Hosp.	Day Care	Indiv. Therapy	Drug	Group	Other**
	23	9	4	29	15	7	11

*Some patients had more than one treatment modality.

**Includes administrative interviews, social casework, and family therapy.

BIBLIOGRAPHY

Annesley, P. Psychiatric Illness in Ado-
    lescent Presentation and Prognosis.
    J. Ment. Sci. 107:268-278, 1961.
Beavers, W. and Blumberg, S. A Follow-up
    Study of Adolescents Treated in an
    Inpatient Setting. *Dis. Nerv. Syst.*
    29:606-612, 1968.
Carter, A. The Prognostic Factors of Ado-
    lescent Psychoses. *J. Ment. Sci.* 88:
    31-81, 1942.
Garber, B. *Follow-up Study of Hospitalized
    Adolescents.* New York, London: Bruner/
    Mazel, 1972.
Gossett, J. and Lewis, J. Follow-up
    Study of Former Inpatients of the
    Adolescent Service, Timberlawn Psy-
    chiatric Center. *Timberlawn Foundation
    Report No. 37, 1969.*
Gossett, J., Lewis, S., Lewis, J.,
    Phillips, V. Follow-up of Adolescents
    Treated in a Psychiatric Hospital: A
    Review of Studies. *Amer. J. Orthopsychiat.*
    43:602-610, 1973.
Hartmann, E., Glasser, B., Greenblatt, M.,
    Solomon, M.H., and Levinson, D.J.
    Adolescents in a Mental Hospital. New
    York: Grune and Stratton, Inc., 1968.
_____, _____, & Herrera, M.A. Adolescent
    Inpatients: Five Years Later. *Seminars
    in Psychiatry.* 1:66-78, 1969.

197

Hollingshead, A.B. and Redlick, F.C.
    Social Class & Mental Illness.   New York:
    York & Wiley, 1958.
King, L. and Pittman, G. A Six Year
    Follow-up Study of Sixty-Five Adoles-
    cent Patients: Predictive Value of
    Presenting Clinical Picture. *Brit. J.
    Psychiat.* 115:1437-1441, 1969.
Levy, E. Long-term Follow-up of Former
    Inpatients at the Children's Hospital
    of the Menninger Clinic. *Amer. J.
    Psychiat.* 125:1633-1639, 1969.
Masterson, J. Prognosis in Adolescent
    Disorders. *Amer. J. Psychiat.* 114:
    1097-1103, 1958.
Myers, J.K., & Bean, L.L. *A Decade Later:
    A Follow-up of Social Class and Mental Ill-
    ness*.   New York, London, Sydney:
    John Wiley & Sons, Inc., 1968.
Pollack, M., Levenstein, S. & Klein, D.
    A Three Year Post-Hospital Follow-up
    of Adolescent and Adult Schizophrenics.
    Amer. J. Orthopsychiat. 38:94-109, 1968.
Warren, W. A Study of Adolescent Psy-
    chiatric Inpatients and the Outcome
    Six or More Years Later: II. The
    Follow-up Study. *J. of Child Psy-
    chology & Psychiatry.* 6:141-160, 1965.

INDEX